One Pogo Jump to Heaven

**A Teenager's Battle with
and Victory over Depression
& A Family's Journey through Grief**

The Prosapio Family

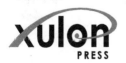

xulon
PRESS

ONE POGO JUMP TO HEAVEN
A Teenager's Battle with and Victory over Depression
& A Family's Journey through Grief
by The Prosapio Family

The book cover was illustrated by Kellie Weber.

Printed in the United States of America.

ISBN 9781498437028

www.xulonpress.com

Table of Contents

Dedication

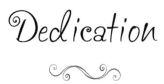

To Wendi Watson, who like Katie had a missionary call to Asia, and to her beautiful family and friends.

To our family, friends, and supporters who have continued to encourage us in our journey. This book is a testament to the love you poured into Katie's life and into each one of us.

Prologue

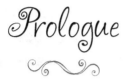

(Written by Katie's Dad, Jerry)

It was a cold, misty, rainy night the evening of March 27, 2006. My wife Pat, son Brian, daughter Laura, and I had just enjoyed a pizza at one of our favorite restaurants. I drove to the neighborhood drug store, and the three of them went in to get some photos developed. The photos were from our recent trip to Rockford, Illinois. They were joyous photos of Laura's spelling bee competition there, along with ones of her older sister, Katie, with her. My thoughts turned to Katie, and I checked my cell phone for any new messages. There were none. I listened to an old message from Katie, as I always saved one to have her voice to hear. However, in the darkness of the car, I inadvertently deleted it. I immediately felt upset to lose the only voice message from her, but as a result, it led me to call her. I rarely called Katie on a weekday night in the seven months that she had been away in the Rockford Master's Commission discipleship program. Saturdays had been our time to talk to each other, and the chance of her picking up the phone during the week was very slim, considering her busy schedule. However, I still wanted to call her to just leave a voice message that her dad was thinking about her and her upcoming missions trip to Vancouver the following Sunday. I was quite amazed when a tired voice answered, and, alas, I was talking with Katie. Realizing I had awakened her, I told her to just go back to sleep. After all, I just wanted to say "Hi" and tell her that I loved her. However, Katie being Katie, she perked up and said, "No, I want to talk with you." She asked me how my day was, and I shared with her that it had been a good day. Katie asked me how she would be able to get cash from her debit card for the upcoming missions trip. As I explained how to do this, I mentioned that I saw her mom, brother, and sister coming back to get into the car. I told her I would put her on the speaker phone so that all four of us could talk with her while driving the five minutes home. She asked her brother Brian how he was doing and, upon hearing that he was teaching and enjoying it, Katie told him she was so proud of him. Her mom and sister Laura said "Hi" and asked if she was excited about her missions trip. They also told her about the photos they had just developed. As I found myself pulling into our driveway at home, I knew it was time to end the call. Surprisingly, I did something I had never done before or since while talking on my cell phone. I told Katie we were in our driveway and getting out of our car to go into the house. I asked, "Katie, would you like to go in the house with us?" She answered, "Yes, Daddy, take me in the house with you!" I entered our home, telling Katie that she was coming in with us. I walked up the six stairs inside, telling Katie that we were going up the stairs together. When I told Katie that we were inside at the top of the stairs by the kitchen, she said that she was happy to be with us. We all told her that we loved her. Katie ended our conversation with the words, "I love you all." Little did I know those words would be the last words I would ever hear my precious nineteen-year-old daughter utter in this life.

Chapter One

The Illusion of Riches

(Written by Katie's Dad, Jerry)

*"For the wages of sin is death, but the gift of
God is eternal life in Christ Jesus our Lord."
(Romans 6:23)*

It was a sunny afternoon in March of 1983 in San
Mateo, California. My wife Pat heard a knock on
the front door and opened it. On the other side of the
screen door stood a man named Frank, who asked if I
was home. Pat responded to him that I was not there but
that she would be hearing from me soon. Frank told Pat
that he was a business acquaintance of mine. He heard
we had an infant son and asked Pat if she could bring
him to the door so he could see him. Wanting to show off

her firstborn, Pat walked to the nursery and brought four-month-old Brian to the door. Frank gazed upon Brian and asked if Pat would give me a message when she next talked with me. He told her to tell me, "Brian has a beautifully shaped head." As Frank said goodbye, it seemed to Pat to be a very strange message to deliver to me.

How does a person go from playing penny-ante poker in third grade to a home visit from the mafia endangering my infant son? My first recollection of my involvement in gambling dates back to when I was nine years old. My friends and I would meet in the basement of the house of my boyhood pal, Marty. We played penny-ante poker after school and on Saturday afternoons. Our parents knew where we were and what we were doing, but they saw very little harm in it. They were just happy that we were not out running around the neighborhood. There were time limits that I was under, as I had to go home to eat dinner, but I noticed even at that age a sense of not wanting to stop playing. There was also an excitement that I felt when I came out a winner.

In the next few years of elementary school, from fourth through eighth grade, I began to pitch coins and look for higher-stakes poker games. I started delivering newspapers in sixth grade and making deliveries for a local butcher shop to get money to gamble. As I looked for poker games, I noticed that kids my age were not willing to risk the amount of money I wanted to gamble.

So, I sought out older kids who liked to gamble and found myself hanging out with them. Rarely did I win playing cards with them, but I did enjoy the feeling of risking and being in games with higher stakes.

In my freshman year of high school, I wanted desperately to make the football team. Despite not having ever played in elementary school, I did make it to the final cut. However, I did not make the team. This rejection led me to search for a way to fit in and feel important while in high school. It was around that time I was approached by someone who asked me to distribute betting parlay cards to the other students. This activity seemed to be just the right fit for me. Other classmates would come to me each week to first get their cards and then, by week's end, to turn in their money to me with their sports picks. I was paid a stipend for how many cards I collected, and I always used that money to play the parlay cards with my picks. I did this for one year, with the risk that if I got caught, I would likely be suspended from high school.

The summer after my high school graduation, my parents took me to the horse racetrack. My parents would go there once a year, and this was my first visit with them. I had my dad place a $2.00 daily double bet for me. That $2.00 bet won and paid $80.00. That first win for me was the start of the next fourteen years of being hooked on horseracing. Later that same summer, I went to the track with some friends and won a perfecta that paid $600.00. I called in sick the next day at work. I went to J.C. Penney's and bought two suits with my winnings, and then I drove some distance to an afternoon racetrack where I proceeded to lose the balance of the $600.00. Those two suits were to be the first and last purchases I would make with any gambling winnings until I quit fourteen years later. Gambling winnings for me were only to be used to continue the action of gambling.

I enrolled in college, and my father was able to get me a good summer job that should have paid for my entire school year. However, due to my gambling, which began to take on another form (betting with a bookie on campus), I always had to borrow money from my parents around the month of April in order to make it through the school year. I began my series of lies by telling them that I miscalculated the cost for my books or tuition and just needed a small loan until I made my first check in the summer, at which time I would pay them back. I went on to graduate from college, and my parents, who wanted to see me get my diploma, never did. I told them another lie that none of my other friends' parents were going to be at the graduation and that the college would be mailing me my diploma. The truth was that there was a big stakes horserace the day I was to graduate. I opted to go to the racetrack instead of my graduation ceremony. I still regret that decision I made.

After college, I found a job in sales for a Fortune 500 Company with good income, benefits, and a company car. However, I was also increasing my betting on sports with the bookies and on more high-stakes poker games. I followed the same pattern I had in my youth, migrating towards those who risked and gambled more. However, the losses continued.

At the age of twenty-three, I found myself in an Army recruitment office. They told me that with my college degree, I could begin as an army officer. I wanted to escape the pressures I was bringing upon myself as a result of gambling. They put the paper in front of me to sign and, with the pen in hand, I told them that I would need to sleep on this decision and would be back the next day. It was that evening that I finally opened up to my dad. He had served in World War II for five years and told me that if I thought I was going to escape gambling by joining the army, I was only kidding myself. He told me there were more poker games in the Army and gave me two suggestions: one, just use will power to stop gambling and call it quits, and two, get my mind on something else—go out and find a good woman. Well, I took one of my dad's suggestions (in addition to not joining the army), and that following week I did meet the girl who God has blessed me with—my wife Pat. However, no amount of willpower could stop the gambling addiction that I was trapped in.

It was around this time I made my first trip to Las Vegas. I went with a group of twenty-one people, twenty men and one woman. The woman was the newlywed wife of one of my friends, and the only way he could go with us was if she went too. We arrived in Las Vegas around noon, and our rooms were not yet ready. The hotel told us we could check our luggage with the employees and go out to gamble and have fun. We could check back with them in a couple of hours to get into our rooms. It was in that short two hours of gambling that I lost all the money I came with. One would think this in itself should have convinced me to never step foot in a casino again; however, while losing my money at the craps table, I witnessed something appealing. One of the craps players was stopping the game and asking the pit boss for chips without having to put up any money for it. He only needed to sign his name on a slip of paper to continue his betting. I asked the player next to me how he was able to do that, and he told me that the gentleman was a high-roller with a line of credit from the casino and did not need to put up money right away like everyone else. I learned that he also got a free hotel room, food, and other compensations due to the amount of money he was gambling. It was at *this* moment that I purposed in my heart that I wanted to one day be like him. This desire to be a high-roller someday would begin my casino addiction. As the Bible says in Proverbs 14:12, "There is a way that appears to be right, but in the end it leads to death."

At the age of twenty-six, I partnered with two other friends to open a business in California. We threw all of our efforts into this business, taking low salaries. I gambled only twice for low dollar amounts that first year. Sales started coming in, and the business was doing well, so we went to Las Vegas to celebrate. It was during that trip that I had a big win and was approached by the casino to open a line of credit and now get a free hotel room, food, and show tickets. I did accept, and now that desire to be high-roller had come to fruition.

On subsequent trips to Las Vegas and Lake Tahoe, I suffered big losses, and now the pressure to sell more and bring more profit to our business increased. My girlfriend Pat, who I had been dating for six years now, gave me the ultimatum to either get married or end our relationship. I was now twenty eight and did not want to lose her, so we wed in August of 1980. She had me promise that there would be no gambling on our honeymoon, so we went to Hawaii, which is still one of two states without legalized gambling (Utah being the other). After four days in Hawaii, I became restless without gambling and convinced her to leave Hawaii to finish our honeymoon in Las Vegas. We flew to Las Vegas and, in less than two days, I lost all our wedding gift money. I did not even have $15 for the cab fare to get my bride to the airport in Las Vegas.

I only had $5 left and watched the meter on the cab as it approached that amount. When it hit $4.90 in the middle of the desert, I told the cab driver to pull over and let us out. I explained that we would walk with our luggage the rest of the way. The cab driver extended us mercy and offered to take us the rest of the way at no extra charge. This ending to our honeymoon was definitely not the way to begin a marriage!

The next two years of our life together were a downward spiral as a result of my gambling. I also started drinking more, using drugs, and viewing pornography. These were carriers that were associated with my gambling. I started playing in all-night poker clubs, as well as betting on sports and horses at the local racetracks. My secret trips to Reno and Las Vegas were becoming more frequent, as I now had entered the desperation phase of my compulsive gambling. The following events were unfolding in my life: daily lying to my wife so as to support my gambling (I took on a spirit of lying), excessive credit card debt (I maxed out numerous credit cards), owing bookies large sums of money, and physical suffering (I saw a doctor three times in one year, with symptoms of high blood pressure and dizziness. I was in need of a root canal and went nine months eating and drinking on one side of my mouth so as to not feel the sensitivity on the problem tooth. The dentist who diagnosed the problem could not believe I went that long when I finally returned to get the work done. He thought that I had paid a better price from another dentist to get it fixed. When my doctor asked if I was under any stress, I could not be honest even with him. The reality was that I was involved in two failing businesses, and I owed many investors and family members. My marriage was one big lie and while I was able to sleep at night, my wife was experiencing a nervous breakdown as a result of financial problems due to my gambling.

As if this was not enough, in desperation to get one big win to solve all of my problems, I turned to the Mafia to get a street loan. My barber at the time also had a severe gambling problem, and he was already indebted into a Mafia loan. He mentioned to me that he could introduce me to them. I was desperate, so I met a man named Frank and took out a loan with them. I lost the entire amount I borrowed in the first three days I had the money. I flew to Las Vegas with bad checks to cash and to one casino where I still had open credit. I left my payment for the Mafia with my barber, and he promised to give it to Frank. When he gambled my payment away that day at a local race track, Frank made a visit to my house.

I called Pat from Las Vegas and lied to her that I was in Los Angeles on business. She shared about my visitor and the message he left for me. I fell silent on the other end and told Pat that I needed to get back to work. I was numb. When I hung up the phone, a voice within me said,

"How much more do you want to take this? You are now jeopardizing your family!" I flew home and would like to say that was the last time I gambled, but it was not. I went one more time to the local racetrack at Bay Meadows in San Mateo. Once again, I lost all of the money I could scrape together prior to going. I came out of the track and got into my car, but I could not turn the key in the ignition. I sat there for a long while and finally uttered eight words that changed my life, "God, I am so sick. Please help me." This cry was from a person who at the moment was not even sure if God would listen or even care.

In my childhood years, I had heard teachings about God and Jesus many times, but I would really only turn to him when I needed a big win on a bet to get out of the mess I was in. Recently, I had felt and experienced many dreams of dying. I knew that my eternal destiny would lead me to Hell. But a wonderful thing happened that late afternoon. God did hear my cry, and He did help me. He led me that week to a Gamblers Anonymous (GA) meeting, where I met a man named Bill who offered several hours of his time to help me. He explained what I needed to do to address my debt problems with those I owed. I did not know at the time, but I later realized how important Bill and the sacrificial time he spent helping me would impact my life. Pat and I soon moved back to Chicago, and she and I continued in a support groups there. We met some Christians in the program who God strategically placed in our lives to share His love with us.

It was on September 19, 1987, at 7:05 p.m., that I received the gift of eternal life by accepting Christ as my Savior. Many things changed in my life. That night he delivered me from a habit of swearing. I still cannot get a swear word past my throat. Pornography that I had hidden in my home was cleaned out that evening. Any desire to gamble was lifted, and I have been free of this addiction since April 1983. Pat and I were blessed with two daughters, whom I like to call miracle children. A marriage that seemingly had little hope of surviving my addictions is today based on trust. God's love truly is faithful, even when the odds seem impossible to overcome.

Chapter Two

Katie's Life

(Written by Katie's Mom, Pat)

"Start children off on the way they should go, and even when they are old they will not turn from it." (Proverbs 22:6)

I was just eight years old and the youngest of four children in my family when I experienced the death of my 45-year-old mother, Catherine. Oh, how I cried out when I learned that on the morning of September 26, 1963, my mom died after a surgery to remove a lobe of her lung due to cancer. While my dad was at the hospital, a parish priest came to our house to tell us the most distressing news a child could imagine. My mom, who would hold me in her lap and care for me, was gone. I remember lying in the hallway of our home, punching the walls and screaming out in sadness and loss. When my mom's suitcase later came home without her, I opened it and held onto her clothing. When I saw an empty gum wrapper from a pack that she had given us just a couple days before her surgery, I wept. Many nights, I would cry myself to sleep. I missed my mom so much.

My father Frank was a tower of strength with an unwavering faith in God. Never once did I hear him speak in anger or despair over losing his precious wife, nor did he seem overwhelmed with raising four children on his own. We were also blessed with an aunt and uncle who never married and who were able to help us with our daily tasks. They showed their love and concern for us children on a regular basis. I had another aunt and uncle with six children of their own who also helped our family and gave us the love we needed. My life without a mom was difficult, but I felt continually nurtured by the adults in my life. With the wonderful, godly example from my dad, aunts, and uncles, I became a person with a smile and a positive outlook on life. I gradually was able to accept what had happened to my family. As a result of my family's tragic experience, we became very close with a special, lasting bond.

When I married Jerry and we started our own family, we named our first daughter Catherine, after my mom. Katie joined her big brother Brian, who was four years old at the time. As a young child, Katie bubbled over with excitement and enthusiasm. She would light up the room with joy and happiness. I remember one time she hugged a friend of mine so tightly that she knocked her down. Thankfully, there were no injuries involved! At the age of ten, Katie began to develop a closeness to God during special services at our church. She would sit by herself in the front row and actively participate in the services. When the worship songs were playing, she would dance before the Lord with delight. When the pastor was speaking, she would write down in her journal every word he spoke. She asked to be "dropped off" at church if we couldn't make the three-times-a-week services. She didn't want to miss any of it. She had a passion for others at a young age and would invite her friends to church. I just loved watching her love her best friend, Jesus.

Katie was well aware of being the middle child in our family. She once remarked that she was the cream in the middle of the Oreo cookie. Katie had an amazing, joyful spirit as a child, and while growing up, she maintained her zest for life. Her big smile and pretty, ocean blue eyes would radiate in any room she entered. She hopped up and down when she was excited.

I loved watching Katie grow and seeing her learn many truths from God's Word. She loved attending Sunday school classes, where she would show me her weekly lesson and tell me all about it. One summer, Katie attended a local Vacation Bible School near our home. She invited so many visitors that week that she won a special award: a beautiful Precious Moments Bible.

Katie loved being in spelling bees while in elementary school. Our family had fun reviewing the spelling lists with her and hearing her spell all of these words (many of which we had never heard before). While in eighth grade, Katie won first place in her regional spelling bee and advanced to the ACSI National Spelling Bee in Washington, D.C. I accompanied Katie on this trip, along with her school principal and eighth-grade teacher. On our first night, we went to Ruth's Chris Steak House. Katie didn't want steak, so she ordered chicken. She commented that this was the most delicious chicken she had ever tasted. Her comment brought a chuckle to us at the table, as the rest of us were enjoying our steaks.

On the night before the spelling bee, we attended a reception at the hotel, where we met other spellers and their families. We enjoyed that evening, as each speller was celebrated for his or her accomplishment to make it to this round of the competition. The next morning, Katie woke up and started to prepare for the spelling bee. As a parent, it was very nerve-racking watching my child walk up to the microphone to spell her assigned words. I felt like my heart was racing each time she received a new word. Katie ended up doing very well, placing 17th in the spelling bee. I was so proud of her efforts.

After the spelling bee and a time of lunch, we hopped onto a tour bus and saw many sites around Washington, D.C. We visited such historic places as the Lincoln Memorial, the Vietnam Memorial, the Thomas Jefferson Memorial, and the Iwo Jima Memorial. The highlight of the tour was visiting Arlington National Cemetery and watching the Changing of the Guard. The top four spellers in the bee presented a beautiful wreath to the Tomb of the Unknown Soldier. It was truly one of the most solemn ceremonies I ever beheld.

One of our family's highlights was going on vacations to Disney World. Katie really loved it there. We would arrive at the entrance of Magic Kingdom, and when the bell rang and the gate opened, Katie would run with Jerry and Brian to ride "Splash Mountain." Laura and I would take our time meeting them after they got off each ride. Katie was fearless when it came to rides (unlike her mother).

Her favorite Disney princess was "Ariel" from "The Little Mermaid." Katie would sing all of the songs from that movie with so much expression. I can't help but think of her whenever I see someone wearing clothing with an image of Ariel on it. Sometimes, I find myself entering The Disney Store to pick up an Ariel figurine, recalling the special moments that we shared together. For a brief moment, I am transported to a time many years ago. It always brings a smile to my face.

Time spent on vacation was so carefree and joyful. We had so many laughs, smiles, and excitement. Jerry and I felt like little kids again whenever we entered the Magic Kingdom. Once, when Katie was running to the top of the stairs of the Cinderella Castle, she stopped, looked right at me, waved, and said, "Come on, Mom!" I now have this image forever in my heart and mind. Someday, I will see her again, as she will be beckoning me to the Heavenly Kingdom.

Chapter Three
The Perfect Season

(Written by Katie's Dad, Jerry)

"Blessed is the one who perseveres under trial because, having stood the test, that person will receive the crown of life that the Lord has promised to those who love him." (James 1:12)

J heard it said in one of my early meetings recovering from gambling that "All the things I thought I would get from gambling, I got from *not* gambling." This truly became a reality in my life as other addictions to drugs and alcohol were supernaturally eliminated from my life. The more I pursued God, the more amazed I became of His doing things in my life that I simply never thought were possible. I was finding for the first time in my adult life that the less control I had over my life, the more freedom God offered me.

It was during this time, after being four years free of gambling, that the next blessing came into my life. That blessing was Catherine Nicole, or as she would soon be known to all, Katie. I was convinced that I was going to have another boy, so when the doctor said I had a baby girl, I was stunned. Upon seeing her and being the first one allowed to hold her, I cried like the baby I was holding.

Pat requested that I stop at a store the following morning before going to the hospital. She asked me to buy a pink bow to put in Katie's brown hair for her trip home. I was tickled pink myself to have the honor and joy of picking out the bow for my baby girl.

From the day she was born, Katie was Daddy's girl. She knew how to get me to do anything for her, and I was putty in her hands. There were only two nicknames that I ever called Katie. One was "Axe," which came from someone else, who called her a "Battle Axe," based on a Biblical passage. The other one, which endeared us to each other and which she loved to be called, was "Sweetheart."

Katie grew up playing three different sports—volleyball, basketball, and softball. Her best ability and talent was in volleyball. However, after eighth Grade, Katie did not want to play it in high school. One thing I learned about Katie was that if she did not have the passion to do something, I could forget about her doing it.

Basketball was something Katie liked to play, but again, after sophomore year in high school, she called it the end of her career. Of the three sports, softball was the one Katie was most passionate about. During a period of eight years, she played on various teams, and I enjoyed being an assistant coach on several of her teams. I liked being an assistant coach for a couple of reasons. First, I did not have to decide which kids started the game, and second, I did not have to worry about bringing the equipment to each game.

I did, however, assume the role of manager (head coach) on two of Katie's teams. One was the Crushers, the first team she played on when she was nine years old. It was very interesting trying to coach girls who had never caught a ball, swung a bat, or knew where to go when I told them to take their position on the field. I really enjoyed coaching Katie's first team, along with the assistance of one of the other moms who helped me. There was such pure joy in watching the young girls laughing, enjoying, and learning how to play, all the while not worrying about who won or lost the game.

The second and last time that I coached Katie was not voluntary on my part. Along with continuing to assist in coaching Katie after her first year, I also helped coach my son Brian in Little League. After a total of about seven years coaching softball and Little League, it was time for me to take a place in the stands with the other parents. I needed a rest and just wanted to watch Katie from the other side of the diamond. We decided to go to a new softball league in a neighboring town. There had been a draft, and Katie was placed on a team called the Bobcats. I drove Katie to her first practice, and there stood all of her teammates and one of the moms—but no coach! The mom went on to explain that the daughter of the head coach had a serious illness, and both of them had to withdraw from the team. She told me that she would assist in any way, but she did not know anything about softball. Her next question was, "Can you coach the team this year?" Everything in me wanted to say no, but what came out of my mouth was the exact opposite. I committed to help out at that first practice and wait to see if another dad showed up and wanted the job. Well, I was given a coach's cap with our team name at the next practice.

Two games into the season, the worst thing that I thought could happen did happen as Katie was making a game-winning play at second base. We were winning 8-7, and with two outs and a runner on first base, the opposing team tried to steal second base. Our catcher threw down to Katie, and the ball and the runner's slide came together at the same time. Katie held onto the ball, and the runner was called out. The game was over, but so was Katie's playing, as her thumb was broken. I remember carrying the equipment bag to the next game and asking God, "What in the world am I doing? Katie is now not even part of the team, and we have another twenty games or so to go!" I remember His answer to me in a still, small voice, "Just keep on going." I kept on going, but even Katie asked if she could stay home, as it was boring for her to merely sit on the bench and not be able to play. I allowed her to stay home, and I reluctantly continued on with the season. However, a strange thing happened as the season continued. We went on to win the rest of our games and ended the regular season with a perfect record. I had never coached or seen a team go undefeated. This winning record led to two occurrences: first, the parents of the other kids loved me and, unlike the other teams I had coached on, I did not receive one negative comment all year; second, I witnessed that as we were entering the playoffs, everyone wanted to beat the Bobcats.

We won our first playoff game by a wide margin and before the second game, Katie's cast was removed, and she was given the "green light" to play again. The semi-final game was close, but we won by a few runs. Katie played, but swinging a bat was difficult for her still tender hand. I was not sure if she should play in the next game: the championship. The game began, and I kept Katie out of the starting lineup. We were winning until the fifth inning when the other team took a one-run lead on us.

In the bottom of the sixth inning, I put Katie in the game, and she came up to bat with runners on first and second. She hit the ball down the right field line for a triple. Both runners scored, and we went on to win the championship and to finish undefeated for the season. That same small voice spoke even louder to me after the celebration and the trophies. "Way to keep going," was the message. I remember expressing to God, "You sure have quite a way at teaching me a lesson in life."

There was just one more thing to do later that week. I found where the original team coach and his daughter lived. I informed Katie that we were going for a ride, and she hopped into the car. She asked me where we were going and what I was carrying in my bag. I told her we were going to visit a father and his daughter. We arrived at their house, and the timing was perfect. The family was in the backyard sitting in lawn chairs as we approached. I introduced ourselves to them, told them how we did that past season, and reached into the bag. We gave my trophy to the young girl who was unable to play that year. Suffice it to say, it was an emotional yet God-ordained way to end a perfect season.

Chapter Four

Depression

(Written by Katie's Dad, Jerry)

"God has delivered me from going down to the pit, and I shall live to enjoy the light of life." (Job 33:28)

It is Labor Day as I write this. One of Katie's favorite adventures to do on Labor Day was to go to the Bristol Renaissance Faire near Kenosha, Wisconsin. Her first time at this event was when Pastor Phil Hahn and his wife Chanda, who Katie loved and served under in Kids' Church, invited her to go with them. They really loved this fair and had some fantastic costumes they would don themselves in each year. Chanda provided Katie an extra costume to wear, and they, along with others whom they invited, headed off for a day at the fair. When Katie returned home, she was full of excitement over all that she had seen and done. She showed me pictures of various performances and people in every type of medieval costume I could imagine.

Before sitting down to write this chapter, I drove Pat, Brian, and Laura to this year's Renaissance Faire. For Laura, this will be her second time there, but for Pat and Brian, it will be their maiden voyage. Once again, Pastor Phil and Chanda have extended the invitation to Laura and have provided her with a costume to wear. I know they miss Katie dearly, but I appreciate seeing how they are being used as extensions of God's love to Laura. I also believe it will be a special day for Pat and Brian, as they spend the day with others who loved and walked with Katie at her final Renaissance Faire. I decided that rather than participate in this year's fair, I would use the holiday to write this chapter about Katie's struggle with and victory over depression.

When Katie was in high school, Pat and I noticed her isolation and her no longer singing the songs that we were used to hearing. She was not the Katie we knew. She would go to her room, lock the door, and want to be alone. She took down her Christian-themed posters and started listening to depressing and hopeless music, music we weren't used to hearing in our home. One day, Pat was cleaning her room and found a suicide letter, in which Katie wrote a goodbye to us and let us know that her depression wasn't our fault.

In that letter, she wrote:

> I'm sorry, I truly am. I'm sorry it had to come to this. Please, no one blame yourselves. It's entirely my fault. I'm too sensitive and love people too much, which has partially led to my downfall. I'm just sick of putting on a façade all the time. I don't want to and can't be happy anymore, and no one wants to hang with the depressed Katie. Everything else running together. I love you all, sincerely and truly.

Katie did not want to live anymore. When Pat and I found this letter, we immediately drove to Katie's high school to pull her out of class to go with us. We drove with Katie a short distance to a local forest preserve, and she wondered and questioned why we were so serious. She asked if someone in our family had died. I parked the car, and Pat showed Katie the letter she had discovered. We asked what was going on in her life that had made her write this suicide note. Katie, who seldom cried up until that moment, broke down in tears and said she could not explain the deep, dark thoughts and emotions she was experiencing. She told us she loved us both so very much, but she could no longer find any joy in her life. We, too, were both moved to tears and after hugging her as tightly as we could, told her that we would be there to love, help, and support her in any way we could. We prayed with her that moment and asked God to protect and watch over her and give us direction as to whom and where to turn.

God heard our prayers and connected Katie to just the right Christian counselor. It was a perfect match, and God used this precious woman to pour new life into Katie. She started taking an anti-depressant medication for the depression, and slowly we began to see visible signs of improvement in her. When Katie went to bed each night, I would try to outlast Katie before she fell asleep. I would pray over her for protection and asked that angels would surround her room. I also found myself to be the first person up in the morning and must admit that as I peeked into her room, I hoped to see that her body still had breath.

One special memory I have during this time was when I asked Katie to come out of her room one night to dance to a song I surprised her with, "Beauty and the Beast." Katie later recounted in a Daddy/Daughter Journal that her fondest memory from her teen years was this dance. She wrote to me, "I cherish this memory because it showed me that I wasn't a burden to you at that time (even though I felt like it). You showed me how much you truly cared about me. It reminded me of the days when I was a little girl and gave me hope that I could be happy again." For Pat and

I, this certainly was a time of great trust that God would watch over Katie day by day. Ultimately, we had to place her in God's hands.

It was about this time that her church youth group was going on a missions trip to Portugal. Katie wrote in her journal that she knew God wanted her to experience this opportunity. Up until this time, only the four of us, along with a couple of close friends, knew about Katie's being on anti-depressant medication. Katie asked us to respect her privacy, so we honored this request. However, on the permission slip to go on the missions trip, she had to list the medications she was currently taking. This meant Katie would need to reveal to her youth pastor that she was experiencing depression. It was a big step for Katie to feel comfortable in her recovery to be able to open up about her depression with another person.

Katie traveled with many of her closest friends on this trip to Portugal, and the experience was truly life-changing. She came back to the States with a renewed sparkle in her eyes that we had not seen in some time. She returned with a passion in her heart and a greater realization of God's work around the world. She wrote, "While [in Portugal], I began to remember my first love. I was able to see first-hand that God is at work everywhere. And through every-one's prayers, God pulled me from the pit of depression." We saw a transformation in Katie, and we knew that she was more excited than ever about serving God with her life.

She also told me she would no longer need to take depression medication. Now you would think that I would take the medication pills and flush them down the toilet at that moment. I didn't, but over the next few months, with the help of Katie's counselor, we saw her weaned from the medication and healed from depression.

On her final Wednesday before leaving for the Rockford Master's Commission program, Katie wanted to share her testimony of freedom from depression with her youth group. She knew this would be the last time she would see them for awhile, and she felt an urgency to share how the Lord had pulled her out of that dark pit of depression. Katie asked me if I would accompany her to church so that I could support her, and I answered that I would come.

The evening right before leaving for church, Katie informed me that she was going to be okay and that she didn't need me to go with her to church. She said the Lord was going to be there for her and asked me to pray with her before leaving for church. When she came home that night, there was a radiant look about her, and she told me she was so happy to be used of the Lord to share her testimony with her friends. She told me that three girls came up to her for prayer after she opened up about her life of depression. They were all suffering from depression and asked Katie to pray with them for God to give them freedom.

Chapter Five

My Two Catherines

(Written by Katie's Mom, Pat)

"But store up for yourselves treasures in heaven, where moths and vermin do not destroy, and where thieves do not break in and steal." (Matthew 6:20)

In Katie's senior year of high school, she finalized plans to go to Rockford Master's Commission (RMC). She had wanted to be a missionary to India since the sixth grade when a missionary to India visited our church and shared about his ministry to young girls who were enslaved in a life of child prostitution. When Katie was in high school, she wrote an article for her school newspaper about children suffering in India. Her article began:

"Most children in America have carefree childhoods. In general, a 10-year-old girl's life is punctuated by trips to the park on hot summer days, birthday parties, and watching Disney movies. Now, picture this scene in India. It's muggy outside. No one else is around as a 10-year-old girl walks home from school, her hair in pigtails. She takes huge steps home because she can't wait to tell her mom that she got an A on her most recent test. Suddenly a man creeps up behind her and renders her powerless. She struggles in his tight grip, but she does not have the strength to resist any longer, and she almost falls limp in his hands. Soon, she is awakened by the sound of automobiles and a bump in the road, unsure of where he could be taking her. And then he leads her to a row of zoo-like cages, locks her up, and leaves her. The other girls look at her with hollow eyes. She's too scared to think of what they are about to say. But they don't have to say anything. She is grabbed by the same dark man, who releases her to a 60-year-old man. She doesn't know what to think as he touches her. And when she is slowly drifting off to sleep that night,

somewhere between reality and uncon-
sciousness, it becomes clear that this won't
be just a one-time occurrence. She is now
destined to be a sexual slave, bound to a
life of prostitution. There will be no more
birthday parties for her. No homecoming
dances or fairy tale romances. Her childhood innocence is robbed, and nothing
can bring it back. This isn't a rare occurrence in India. 'Every day, about 200 girls
and women in India enter prostitution, and
80 percent of them against their will. At the
current rate of growth by 2025, one out of
every five Indian girls will be a child prosti-
tute,' according to Save the Children (**www.
savethechildren.in**)."

The nine-month discipleship program at RMC would
help Katie to accomplish her dream to go to India and
rescue girls who were trapped as sex slaves.

Right before leaving for RMC, Katie blessed each of
us with a personal handwritten note. The note she wrote
to me was so precious, and it gave me much hope. Katie
told me that she liked the way I cared for others and said
that I was storing up treasures in Heaven that would last
forever. She thanked me for being her mom and caring for
her from infancy. Katie was so excited when she left for

Rockford, and I was so happy for her that I didn't shed a tear. I knew she was exactly where God wanted her to be.

The last time I saw Katie was ten days before she went to be with the Lord. We had a special two days with Katie as we were in Rockford for our youngest daughter Laura's regional spelling bee. The Lord gave me such a peaceful memory the night Katie stayed with us at the hotel. I slept in the same bed with Katie and woke up several times during the night to the sight of her sleeping sweetly and her long, curly, brown hair. I will treasure that memory forever. As I said goodbye to Katie, she gave me a big bear hug and exclaimed, "I want to go with you!" I said, "It won't be much longer until you are done and will be coming home." If I knew that would be my last hug, I would have made it last longer, and I would have held her tighter.

I worked at my job as a Neonatal Intensive Care Unit (NICU) nurse on March 28, 2006, with two other nurses in our unit. I recall it as a fun day, being more lighthearted than usual. We worked with a funny neonatologist, and interestingly, we sang, "Que será, será—whatever will be, will be—the future's not ours to see—que será, será." Who would have known that Katie had already passed into eternity an hour after I had started working?

After work, I drove home and sat in our living room. Jerry and I were deciding on what to have for dinner when we heard an unexpected knock at the door. We opened the door to behold Katie's youth pastor and another church member. A serious look was displayed on their faces as they assertively asked us to walk downstairs and to sit down on our couch. They explained to us that Pastor Jeremy DeWeerdt (the director of RMC) called, and that Katie and her classmate Wendi had been involved in a car accident. After they uttered these words, we knew that she was no longer with us. Our precious daughter, along with her good friend Wendi Watson, had left this earth forever. We cried and hugged each other tightly, shocked and in disbelief.

Almost immediately, our house filled with family and friends. Katie's former children's pastor, John Schwider, ran into our house with tear-stained eyes, not believing what had happened. Another friend walked into the house angrily, questioning why this had happened. At the time I learned of Katie's death, I immediately knew she was experiencing Jesus and Heaven in all of its glory. As I was pondering this reality, our former pastor's wife led us all in a time of singing before the Lord. We even listened to Katie's song, "Remembering the Persecuted." (You may listen to this song at: www.katiescomfort.org.) We received so much comfort that night, knowing the Holy Spirit was truly in our midst. His comfort rested on our hearts as we praised Him during that time of great pain.

God was so evident in the preparation of Katie's wake and funeral. Our pastor and his wife met us at the funeral home and sat with us in the conference room to make all of the arrangements. The funeral directors handled everything with such dignity and respect. One special memento that the directors were able to salvage from the fiery accident was a woven rainbow-colored necklace that Laura had made for Katie before she had left for RMC.

On March 31st, the day of the wake, we had an hour to be alone with Katie before everyone else came. We stood beside a closed white casket. A picture of her rested on top of the casket, as well as a Bible that was opened up to a passage that was very meaningful to her, Romans 12. The room was filled with flowers sent by loved ones and posters of Katie with family and friends. We also displayed the final note that Katie sent to us, saying, "Thanks Mom and Dad for sending me to Master's."

Many individuals lined up to say goodbye to Katie and to pay their respects to us. The wake began at 2:00 p.m. and lasted until 10:45 p.m. The line extended all around the funeral home, into a vacant room, and even outside. It reminded me of a line for a rollercoaster. In this line, people talked to each other and shared memories of Katie. One of the moments I remember the most was when Katie's counselor approached us, who we had not seen for some time. She was visibly pregnant with her first child. She said she didn't plan to have children because she thought they would become very difficult to raise during their teenage years. She had counseled many teens with difficult situations, including rebellion. She said getting to know Katie and witnessing her recovery had changed her mind in favor of having children. It was such a blessing to see and hear this testimony of how God placed Katie and her counselor together to help one another.

On April 1st, the day of Katie's funeral, I went outside to get our neighborhood newspaper. On the front page was the headline, "Spiritual teen dies in fiery crash." The article tenderly shared about Katie, her compassion and love for others, and her dream as a young girl to become a missionary to India. After reading this article, I felt such joy for having been her mom. As I got ready for the service, which I knew was going to be a celebration of Katie's life, I put on a black blazer with small pink rosettes on it, a pastel pink shirt, and a black skirt. My precious friends supplied me with this outfit, as they knew I could not shop for clothes. As I walked into our church, the first people I saw were my brother, his wife, and my niece and nephew. We hugged for a moment, and I said to them with a smile, "We are going to celebrate Katie's life today." I felt no despair or sadness at the time. God was comforting me supernaturally at this most difficult time in my life.

Before the service started, we were greeted by all of Katie's classmates at Rockford Master's Commission, about 130 of them in all. They hugged us, cried with us, and told us how much Katie had meant to them. We were overjoyed at the love we felt from them. We then sat down in the front row of the church. The service was absolutely beautiful and was so honoring to our precious daughter. Several pastors, along with one of the pastor's wives who was a personal mentor to Katie, spoke about her life and the impact she had made on others. Two of Katie's closest friends stood together to share about Katie and the memories and love that they shared. There were funny familiar stories that brought much laughter, as well as stories that we had never heard before that brought an increased sense of wonder for the life we had been blessed to know.

Pastor Jeremy DeWeerdt from RMC said Katie was the most "alive" person he had ever met. He presented us with a beautiful brown chest filled with letters to our family from the RMC students, giving their condolences and sharing memories of Katie. This act of love touched us in amazing ways. Whenever I miss Katie and want to be uplifted, I read one of those Heaven-sent letters. This was another way the Lord comforted me, both then and now. Later in the service, Katie's song, "Remembering the Persecuted" was played. Her voice echoed in the sanctuary, and it felt as if she was right there with us. She wrote this song to encourage missionaries and Christian believers in persecuted areas around the world. The gospel message was also shared, and fifteen people raised their hands to commit their lives to Jesus Christ. Katie had always prayed for her family and friends to come to know Jesus in a personal way. That day her prayers were answered.

When we arrived at the cemetery to say our goodbyes, the tone was more somber. It was our final physical separation from Katie. A friend played "Amazing Grace" on the bagpipes. Pastor John Schwider read a passage of scripture and said a prayer that comforted us. Jerry also shared a thought from Hebrews 12:1, that Katie was now in a great cloud of witnesses, encouraging us to finish our race of life. We then returned to the church for a luncheon graciously provided by our church family. The RMC students ate their meal while we were at the cemetery, as they had to return to Rockford, IL, for Wendi's funeral later that day. Our pastor ordered enough food for 200 people. However, 130 students had just eaten, and the ladies who prepared the food were concerned that there would not be enough food for the rest of us. So, the ladies prayed for there to be enough food. As they reached down for more food, they observed a miraculous occurrence. There was always another box to serve! In fact, there was enough food for them to take home to their families and to serve to another group of Master's Commission students coming from Arkansas the following day. What an awesome God we serve!

In the days that followed Katie's wake and funeral, I felt as though I was walking through the valley of the shadow of death, as it says in Psalm 23:4. The hardest moments were looking through Katie's belongings and clothing. I felt as if my heart was broken. I cried as I clung to her clothes, remembering what she looked like in them. As I emptied her gym bag, I saw an empty gum wrapper. All of a sudden, I was a child, holding my mother's dress and seeing an empty gum wrapper in her suitcase. Both of my Catherine's were gone. More than ever, I needed God's comfort, and He was truly there. He saw every tear I cried, and as it says in Psalm 56:8, all of these tears were collected in a bottle.

Chapter Six

Sibling Love

(Written by Katie's Brother, Brian, and Sister, Laura)

"Keep on loving one another as brothers and sisters." Hebrews 13:1

Katie was blessed to have an older brother, Brian, and a younger sister, Laura, as siblings. Brian was four years older and Laura was seven years younger. Brian and Laura have wonderful memories of their sister they will share in the following pages.

Brian

One of my first memories as a child was when Katie came home from the hospital after her birth. I can still remember her lying in her basinet. As I looked at her, I remember feeling a sense of responsibility, as much as a four-year-old boy could have. I was now a big brother and had to do what I could to protect her. As we grew up together, I tried to fulfill this personal goal. At the same time, Katie and I had a lot of fun together! We played games that we made up, such as wrapping ourselves in a blanket and rolling off the bed laughing and screaming. We also loved to watch kids' shows and cartoons together, including just about everything on Nickelodeon. We loved to spend time with each other. We both attended a Christian school and learned about God and His plan for our lives. This knowledge gave us a sense of purpose for our lives and would later help us to weather the storms that came our way.

When Katie was ten years old, our church began to experience a wonderful move of God, accompanied by amazing times of prayer. Katie and I would pray together at home on a regular basis. She once wrote to me in a note:

> Dear Brian, I love you so much!!! You are a great friend. I was wondering, would it be okay if we had an overnight together sometime? And, let's have more prayer meetings together, even if we just pray the Lord's Prayer. Let's start praying for those who don't know Jesus. Let's surprise Mom

and Dad sometime and give them dinner.
Mom and Dad will love that. Well, is high
school hard? You are a great brother. Love,
your pal, Katie.

I'm not sure if we ever did make dinner for our parents,
but I do remember our prayer times. This letter shows
Katie's heart for God and others, even at a young age.

When Katie began high school and I began college,
we did not see each other as much but we still found ways
to keep in touch. In a way, our relationship grew deeper.
We would have long conversations about different things
on our minds. In the process, we shared some laughs and
learned from each other. Most of the time we had these
conversations in Katie's room before she fell asleep.
There was something peaceful about these conversations. I believe it was because Jesus, the Prince of Peace,
was in the room with us. I would encourage siblings, even
when they are older, to continue to talk to each other and
learn from one another.

One other way Katie and I grew close to each other
was through our summer vacations. There is something
about sharing a hotel room that brings a family together;
there is no place to hide or do your own thing. You are
forced to experience life together. That can be a good
thing or bad thing. It can be good because you spend
more time together, but it can be bad because you might

get on each others' nerves. However, I believe the good outweighs the bad as wonderful memories are formed. Katie and I had so many wonderful memories together as we were blessed to spend some of our summers at Wisconsin Dells, Indiana Beach, and Disney World. Our first time at Disney World, we stayed at a hotel that had many programs for kids, as well as a mascot named Max who roamed around the grounds greeting everyone. Little did we know that he also visited the guests' rooms and tucked in kids at nighttime. Needless to say, we were quite surprised when he appeared in our room to tuck us in! At the end of the trip, Katie got a stuffed animal of Max, which she slept with every night at home. I love to look at the pictures from these vacations, as well as the camcorder footage that was taken. It brings me back to another time and place and makes me feel warm inside, even though she is no longer with me. I would encourage families to make time in their busy schedules for vacations, even if they are short in length or are close to home, as wonderful memories can be made.

When Katie left for Rockford Master's Commission in the fall of 2005, there was a sadness in my soul. In fact, I was sad for about a week. I guess you could say I was grieving a loss. In a way, it prepared me for truly losing her in the spring of 2006. However, I did see her a few times in between, and our times together were rich. I remember sitting in church together and watching our sister Laura become an Honor Star in the Missionettes program at our church. I also remember Christmas morning and her idea for our family to share communion together. The last memory I have of Katie was at the Museum of Science and Industry in Chicago on New Year's Day in 2006. It was a family tradition of ours to go to the museum on New Year's Day. On this particular day, we were just about to leave the museum when Katie took me by the hand; and we walked, hand in hand, out of the museum. We did not share many words that day, but we did share our love for each other. It was the last outing that we would have together. She returned to Rockford a few days later.

Although we did not see each other again, we did have some beautiful conversations on the phone. Our family talked to her the night before she went to be with the Lord. We had her on the speaker phone, and we all talked together. The one thing she told me was that she was proud of me. I had just started my teaching career and was a substitute teacher at the time. Her words of encouragement helped me to continue on, despite a challenging substitute teaching position. Now, I am in my eighth year as a teacher, thanks to the Lord and to my sister's early encouragement to continue on.

The moment I heard that Katie had passed away, two emotions flooded my soul. One was of shock, not understanding how this could happen. The other was one of comfort, knowing that my sister was in the presence of

God. As time went on, I learned just how much Katie wanted to be with her Lord in Heaven. She had dreamed about the day she would meet Jesus face to face. And God ultimately gave her the desire of her heart. Although her life on this earth was short, it was an abundant life. As Jesus said in John 10:10, "I have come that they may have life, and that they may have it more abundantly." That is God's plan for our lives.

As time went on after this loss, I found comfort through the many people who visited our house and gave us meals. They were an expression of God's love to us. I also found help by going to a Christian counselor and talking through the emotions I was feeling. I would encourage anyone, if they are going through a situation that is too difficult for them to face alone, to talk to someone else about it. Help is available from God and from other people.

Now, nine years later, I look forward to the moment when I will see Jesus face to face, and be reunited with my sister and other relatives who have gone before me. What a wonderful moment that will be! In the meantime, I want to be about my Father's business and doing what He wants me to do with my life. He has a plan for each and every one of us on this earth. Katie fulfilled God's plan for her life. Do you know God's plan for your life? If you do not know where to begin, it is as simple as **A-B-C**. The Bible says that, "All have sinned and fall short of the glory of God" and that "the wages of sin is death, but the

gift of God is eternal life through Jesus Christ our Lord."
Once you accept this basic truth, all that you have to do is:

A. **Admit you are a sinner.** "There is no one righ-
   teous, not even one...for all have sinned and fall
   short of the glory of God." Romans 3:10, 23. (Also
   see Romans 5:8 and 6:23.) **Ask God's forgiveness.** "Everyone who calls on the name of the
   Lord will be saved." Romans 10:13.

B. **Believe in Jesus** (put your trust in Him) as your
   only hope of salvation.

   "For God so loved the world that he gave his
   one and only Son, that whoever believes in
   him shall not perish but have eternal life."
   John 3:16. (Also see John 14:6.) **Become
   a child of God by receiving Christ.** "To
   all who receive him, to those who believed
   in his name, he gave the right to become
   children of God." John 1:12 (Also see
   Revelation 3:20.)

C. **Confess that Jesus is your Lord.** "If you confess
   with your mouth, 'Jesus is Lord,' and believe in
   your heart that God raised him from the dead, you
   will be saved." Romans 10:9 (Also see verse 10.)

When you take these simple steps, you become a part of the family of God, and He places His Holy Spirit in you to lead and guide you. Other good steps would be to talk to God on a regular basis in prayer and to find a church congregation where His Word, the Bible, is proclaimed. It is also good to share this good news that you have found with others in your life, so that they too can find out God's plan for their lives. If this is a new step for you, and you have made a decision to accept Jesus as your Lord and Savior, let me be the first to welcome you into the family of God! If you have any questions, please do not hesitate to contact us at **info@katiescomfort.org**.

Laura

Katie came into my life on March 12, 1994, the day that I was born. I love watching a home video recording of her cradling me for the first time at the hospital. She was smiling, and I cooed. Our bond formed at that very moment. She imparted her influence on me while I was growing up, whether or not she knew it. That influence she had on me changed my life for the good, and because of her, I will never be the same.

Katie and I were typical sisters. We got into our little squabbles once in a while, but our love for each other never faded. And both of us knew that was true. She was seven years older than me, so our interests differed as we grew up. As a teenager, she was interested in her guitar and hanging out with her friends, while I was a child interested in playing with Barbies and watching cartoons. Although we had those little differences, our common bond was love.

Katie had this way about her of making situations humorous. One day I invited my best friend Anna over to my house, and we were just sitting on our living room couch and talking. Katie had the bright idea to grab jumbo marshmallows out of the bag, stuff them into her mouth, and chase me and my friend around the house. We screamed as she rampaged about like a gorilla on the loose. My crazy big sister surely knew how to brighten up somebody's day.

Another time, Katie had plans to go out with some friends. I knew that I hadn't gotten to see her much lately, and she recognized the same fact. As a result, she decided to change her plans and drove me to Baskin Robbins where we got ice cream (Katie's favorite treat). We sat outside on a concrete curb for a long time, just talking and laughing until the sunset subsided to nightfall. It touched me so much that Katie cared about my awkward adolescent life. From taking me to movies I wanted to see to having sleepovers with me in my bed— we enjoyed the time we spent together.

One summer night I was having trouble falling asleep. As I looked out my bedroom door, I saw a light coming from upstairs. I knew somebody must be awake. So I resolved to check things out. I found my sister upstairs taking her contacts out and looking pretty tired. I told her about my hard time getting to sleep, and she said she would come down to my room right after she finished getting ready for bed. So I walked downstairs and rested in my bed until Katie came down to my room. She plopped down next to me, and we started talking. I asked her questions pressing in my mind about the Holy Spirit and my relationship with God. She greatly helped me that night by giving me her answers to my questions. I appreciated her insights, and especially her life experiences that she shared to demonstrate to me God's faithfulness. I distinctly remember her telling me, "Whenever you have trouble falling asleep again, I'm here for you." And I thought to myself, *Wow! My sister is the best.*

The times that I hold most dear with my sister were when she mentored me in my faith. She was on the worship team for youth group at church, so she had a book filled with chord charts for worship songs that would frequently be played at services. One night when I was sitting in our family's living room, she sat down next to me and started playing worship songs. She took requests, and I listened. Apparently, she wasn't satisfied with my just listening. She asked me to start worshipping God with her. And I thought to myself, *Wow! I'm so thankful my sister challenges me to love the Lord more.* That night, we formed our own little worship service with songs that connected us with the heart of God and with each others' hearts.

Before Katie left for Rockford, she volunteered as a kids' church leader at church; I was so proud to have my sister as a leader. She acted out lessons to us kids that were part of the curriculum for kids' church. But, of course, Katie had a way of making the lessons her own—and especially entertaining.

In kids' church, we had some very meaningful times of worship to the Lord. One song entitled "I Love You Lord" was especially powerful when all the little children joined with one voice praising Jesus. On one Sunday in particular, I spotted Katie with a tear running down her cheek. Katie told me how much she could feel the Lord's presence in kids' church, especially when we sang that song. She had a compassionate heart for people of all ages. From kids, to her own teenage friends, to adults, and to the elderly, Katie brought God's overflowing joy.

During that summer, Katie felt a prompting by God to visit a local nursing home to minister to the elderly. She felt a burden for them after she woke up one morning and felt that she should go visit with them by singing and playing her guitar. She printed off some lyrics to church hymns, and my mom drove me and her to a nearby nursing home (I decided to tag along to see what my sister had up her sleeve). As we entered the building, we found a person who worked there, and he directed Katie to the room where she would play. As we wandered into the room, there was an audience of elderly people waiting for my sister's ministry. She pulled up a chair in the center of the room, and my mom and I sat to the side. She started singing and playing her guitar. She sang hymns such as "In the Garden" and "He Keeps Me Singing." I could tell by the faces of the people that they were touched. Some even tried singing along with her. One man had a set of maracas and was cheerily playing his instrument to the beat—or at least attempting to! I could tell that Katie shone Christ's love, especially when she knew she was doing what God wanted her to do—a leading of the Holy Spirit to use her gifts to bless others.

A few weeks later, Katie felt God prompt her to go back to the nursing home a second time. I decided to tag along again with her to help in any way I could. Katie again ministered with what she did best—worshipping the Lord with all of her heart. As she neared the end of her ministry that morning, she asked me to come to the middle of the room to sing with her. I was hesitant, but somehow Katie, with her bright blue eyes and convincing smile, persuaded me to join her. She had me sing "Jesus Loves Me" along with her. As my nervousness melted away in my worship, I realized how fulfilling it was to praise God and minister to others. Katie helped to teach me that giving to others helps me to live as Christ lived.

About a week before Katie left for Rockford, she left each of my family members a personal letter on the kitchen counter communicating her love for us. This was a great surprise to all of us. As I opened my letter, I read:

Dear Lil' Sis-

I love you so much! I'm sorry we haven't gotten to spend that much time together lately…but that's gonna change.

I don't know if you recall something about a (what was the word…hmm…) Oh I remember, DATE!

We're going on one, you see! To Pizzeria UNO (w/ cute waiter to get a <u>cookie</u> sundae/ bowl/etc.) to Hollywood Park, to wherever else your lil' heart desires.

You pick the date. I'll be there.

I've been busy sleeping but not anymore. You've got Katie back! Full throttle! Bigger and better than ever! Can you handle this? (Best for ages 11 & up)-That's you!

So are you excited about school? I'm gonna pluck your eyebrows. [This was something she loved to do for some reason] I hope it doesn't hurt too much. We can go for a walk too and talk about stuff. It will

be a lot of fun. We can even watch (drum
roll, please) Father of the Bride 2! Hooray.
I love you lil' sis. If I have any more clothes,
I know who to give them to! Love, Katie

I loved the times we walked around the neighborhood
and just talked about life. She asked me about school
and church and miscellaneous happenings in my life. My
fondest memory of her was our infamous "date" before
Katie left for Rockford Master's Commission (RMC). As
an opening ceremony to our little "date," we watched a
movie called *A Little Princess*, based on the novel written
by Frances Hodgson Burnett. This movie is about a little
girl named Sarah who has lost her mother and lives with
her father. Her father goes off to war, and Sarah doesn't
know if she'll ever see her father again. Before he departs,
the two of them have a tender moment together of saying
good-bye. Her father gives her a doll named "Emily," and
he tells Sarah that whenever she hugs Emily, she'll really
be getting a hug from him. He goes off to war, and the
little girl holds onto the love of her father, symbolized by
the doll he left for her. This movie really impacted me,
especially the part about Sarah receiving a hug from her
father every time she hugged the doll he had given her.

For the rest of our day together, we took a trip to the
thrift store where we tried on wacky clothes. I remember
trying on colorful dresses and pajamas and hearing what

Katie thought about each item I tried on. After the thrift store, we walked to a favorite shopping center near our house. I think she purposely led us on the long way so that we could talk more. We arrived at a Hallmark store and glanced at various items, but one in particular caught my eye. I spotted a pink elephant stuffed animal with blue ears and a blue tail named "Winks." Katie apparently saw my fascination with the elephant, and I saw her pick up the elephant and carry it around the store. I began to wonder why she was holding it. As the time neared for us to leave the store, she approached the checkout counter with the stuffed elephant and bought it for me. I was touched she did this for me (especially realizing she was the typical college student with a tight budget). We walked out of the store toward Pizzeria UNO, which is a Chicago-style type grill and also our favorite place to eat together. We started talking about her preparation for Master's Commission, and she said she wanted to get me "Winks" the elephant so that I could remember her. *"How could I ever forget Katie?"* I thought. She stressed that I would probably forget her when she was gone at school (this makes me laugh because not a day has gone by that I have been unaware of her love). I told her, "Katie, I will never forget you." There was a silence as I began thinking about the movie we had watched the night prior. I asked Katie, "Could Winks be like Emily in *A Little Princess*? Whenever I give him a hug, I'll really be hugging you." She liked the idea, and we resolved that whenever I hugged my elephant, I'd really be sending a hug to my big sister.

While at Pizzeria UNO, we split a Deep Dish Sundae (a giant chocolate chip cookie topped with ice cream and whipped cream). And let me tell you, we gobbled that thing up!

Katie had her camera flip phone with her, and we decided to take snapshots of each other in the booth we were sitting in. That was really fun because when we took pictures of the both of us together, sometimes neither I nor Katie got in the frame of the picture. Apparently we had really bad aim.

We ended that "date" with much laughter as we walked back home. That day was an incredible bonding experience, and I carried it with me for the months she went away to Rockford.

The weekend for her to go to Rockford drew near, and before I knew it, my family was driving her to Master's Commission. I was extremely sad but also extremely happy for her. I knew Katie was supposed to be there, and I couldn't do anything but rest in the knowledge that God had her there for a purpose. When we arrived at Rockford, we drove her to her townhouse, where she was to live for the upcoming months. We unpacked her belongings, and we brought them up to her room. Let me tell you, Katie was not a light packer! Trip after trip, we carried her belongings from the car, up the stairs, and into her room. She made her bed, and we organized her closet until the room was ready. She met with the four girls she would be staying with and seemed very excited.

The weekend passed quickly, until it was finally Sunday, the day we had to let our Katie go for the first time. We attended church with her at Rockford First that morning, and after the church service, we dined at a barn-themed restaurant. It finally sank in that my Katie was going to leave me for a few months, and I was so distressed. She consoled me, though, and she comforted me as only she could do, assuring me we'd see each other before we knew it. We had an enjoyable time eating together, and after we were done, the time came for us to bring her back to her new "home," where we were to say our good-byes. She gave us all hugs and kisses, and we told her that we loved her. I always enjoyed the phone calls we received from Katie while she was away, but nothing compared to the times when we visited her and she visited us.

About six months later in March of 2006, I competed in a spelling bee in Rockford. As a result, we got to visit with Katie while we were up there. We met for lunch at Applebee's, and Katie and I split a delicious dessert (a caramel apple sundae) to celebrate our birthdays. The following day was St. Patrick's Day (the day of the spelling bee competition). With God's help, I qualified to advance on to Nationals that upcoming May. When Katie heard the news, she blurt out, "What! You're so young!" That made me smile. She advanced to Nationals in Washington, D.C., five years prior, and I looked up to her for that.

We ate a St. Patrick's Day lunch at Cracker Barrel, and headed to the hotel where my dad, mom, and I were staying. She decided to sleep over in the hotel with us that night, and she shared a bed with my mom while I slept on the floor. She called me up to sleep in the bed with her and my mom, but I fell off twice from lack of space! Dismayed, I decided to just stay on the floor. But Katie called me back up again to have some more bonding time before I fell asleep. I eventually did go to sleep on the floor, though (thankfully it wasn't *too* bad). We all had a decent sleep, and in the morning, my dad brought McDonald's pancakes into our hotel room where Katie and I feasted. I remember she wore pajamas with sheep on them, and I made up a song about them that I sang to her all morning.

My parents and I got ready to leave for our journey home, and my mom and dad started packing up the car with all of our belongings. For a time, it was just me and my sister in the hotel room lying on the bed. We lay there just staring into each others' eyes and smiling at each other. She broke the silence by starting to talk to me about the topic of God's grace. She stressed that I learn to understand what grace truly is. She explained to me that we don't have to earn our salvation by obeying laws.

Jesus fulfilled the law when He died on the cross for our sins, and because of His sacrifice, we are made whole and clean. His mercies are there for us every morning, and we don't have to live in condemnation. I was having trouble with guilt at that time in my life, and Katie helped set me on a path that would lead me to begin comprehending God's grace. This was our last conversation together face to face, and it will always live on in my heart. I can still sense the closeness of her freckled face and her brown spiral curls resting upon her shoulders. In that moment, her mouth spoke wisdom, and her eyes searched for my understanding.

The time came for us to leave Rockford. We all walked outside to the snowy parking lot to say our good-byes, and Katie went back into the hotel room to take a nap before checking out. For some reason, we forgot an item in the hotel room, and my mom had to go back. I decided to tag along so I could say good-bye to my sister one more time. My mom found what she forgot, said good-bye to Katie, and exited the room while I lingered with Katie for a few more short moments before I had to leave. I remember her tossing me on the bed and tickling me. She said, "I love you, Little Lötte" (Little Lötte was what she called me), we embraced tightly, and then I walked out of the hotel to join my dad and mom outside for our departure. That was the last time I saw my big sister here on this earth, and I will cherish it for as long as I live.

Chapter Seven

Katie's Journal Entry Fulfilled

(Written by Katie's Dad, Jerry)

"Very truly I tell you, unless a kernel of wheat falls to the ground and dies, it remains only a single seed. But if it dies, it produces many seeds." (John 12:24)

When Katie was sixteen years old, she gave me a Daddy/Daughter journal for Father's Day. It was divided into two sections, with both of us having to respond to questions about our relationship with each other. The questions were quite emotional for me to answer, even while Katie was here on the earth with me. It asked such questions as, "What was it like to hold your daughter for the first time?"

I knew that for a person like me who had never journaled before, this was going to take some time and effort on my part. Katie would periodically ask me, "Daddy, did you finish your portion of the journal?" My response would always be, "Do you want the book back first to do your part?" Her answer was always no. She would say, "Daddy, you do your part first, then give it to me." She really knew her dad when it came to my writing ability. (She would be amazed to see me taking on my writing portion of this book that you are now reading!)

Katie's eighteenth birthday was the perfect day to have my portion done to give it to her. You should have seen the joyous look on Katie's face when I gave her the journal! Later that night, after reading some of my entries, she came to me, and with a familiar hug (this time a little bit tighter), she told me that this was the best present I had ever given her. My immediate response back to her was, "When are you going to finish your portion and give it back to me?" Having taken two years to do my part, she just gave me one of those looks, as we knew each other all too well.

God had placed a special dream in Katie's heart. Pat wrote earlier that when Katie was in sixth grade, a missionary to India came to our church and shared about his ministry to young girls who were imprisoned in a life of child prostitution. Upon hearing that message, Katie's future plans were eternally impacted. She attended a summer church youth camp later that year and came home telling us how the Lord had called her to be a missionary to India. Her eyes and expression were filled with anticipation as she shared this revelation with us. Pat and I had heard many amazing testimonies from visiting missionaries of their call to serve God overseas. It was now for the first time, even at Katie's early age, that God showed me He wanted my young daughter for His service. I was unaware of all of the ways this could be accomplished, but Pat, Brian, Laura, and I always supported Katie in the call on her life.

The day we helped move Katie into the townhouse she would be sharing with four other girls in Rockford, she whispered in my ear before saying goodbye, "Daddy, there is a surprise present I have for you under my mattress when you get home." I gave her one more big kiss and hug, thanked her for the present, and told her I would look for it when I got home. I was sure it was the Daddy/Daughter journal, because I knew my daughter. However, I did not lead on to her of my inclination of her gift under her mattress.

We called Katie later that evening to see how she was doing. (In truth, we cried upon getting home and missed her greatly already!) Right away, Katie asked me, "Daddy, did you find your surprise?" I said I sure did (again, playing out my part as acting very surprised). She then asked me, "Did you read everything I wrote to you?" I told her that I could only read one page due to the emotion of the day. I shared with her that this was going to take some time to read fully, as it was so beautiful and I wanted to savor each entry she wrote. I knew that my response was okay with my Sweetheart.

There was one question and response in the journal that still amazes me to this day. Katie was asked, **"What would you like to do with your dad later on in your life?"** Katie's response was for me to one day come visit her in India. She said she wanted me to see her world and where God had called her to serve Him. Little did I know that God would answer this dream in a way only He could orchestrate.

On June 28, 2008, I stood at a dedication ceremony for the opening of the first Teen Challenge Center in Cambodia (www.tccambodia.com). Pastor Jim Lowans and his wife, Kathie, who were Katie's first children's pastors, were asked to oversee the building of this center for young men addicted to drugs. When Pastor Jim came to Katie's funeral and learned of her desire to serve the Lord in Asia, he and Kathie felt the Lord call them to name this center in Cambodia "Katie Hall." Today, it houses those who are being set free from drugs and, more importantly, who are coming to a knowledge of Jesus Christ. The reality that I was standing a few countries away from India filled me with extraordinary emotions. I sensed that not only did God know when He wanted to call Katie home to Heaven, but that He also saw me standing on that Cambodian property one day.

I have come to see that God views time so much differently than we do, as He is the Alpha and the Omega and knows the beginning from the end of life. That day in Cambodia, I realized that truth and found peace in it.

Before going on this trip, I felt the Lord wanted me to bring something of Katie's to leave in Cambodia. I found some extra wheat stalks that had been laid on Katie's casket at her wake and funeral, and I decided to bring those with me. The last thing I did before leaving "Katie Hall" was crush and spread the wheat across the front of the property. Pastor Jim and his wife Kathie stood next to me as I prayed that there would be new life produced in the young men and in the soil at "Katie Hall." There had been no vegetation up to that day, and the land was very barren. The people in the area believed the land was cursed.

However, in the years since, I am happy to report that many lives have and are continuing to be transformed, and the land has produced many wonderful crops to sustain the work of "Katie Hall." I thank God for making Katie's journal entry a reality.

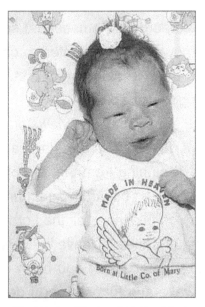

First Baby Photo of Katie. Made in Heaven, now her home.

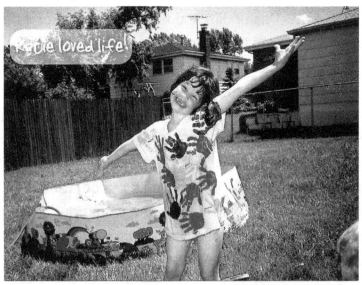

Childlike Joy. Although taken at a very early age, this picture really describes Katie.

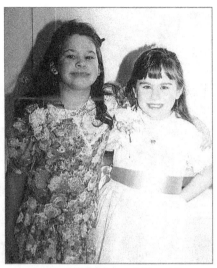

Buddies. Her closest friend from infancy was Bethany, whom she described in her "Heaven Letter."

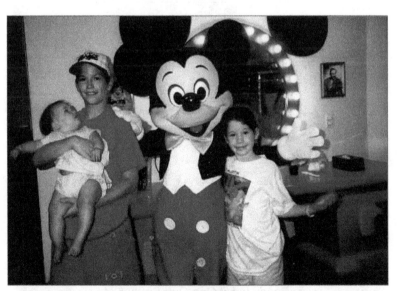

Magic Kingdom. Some of our most precious memories were at Disney World. Here's Brian holding Laura, and Katie smiling with Mickcy.

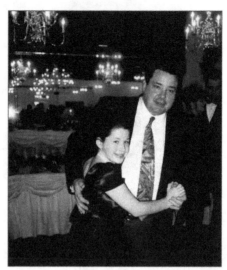

Katie as Junior Bridesmaid. Special dance and just warming up for yearly Daddy-Daughter dances to follow.

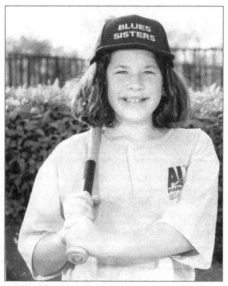

Ready to Hit One Out! Softball at an early age. She loved to play this game, and we met many great people on the various teams she played on.

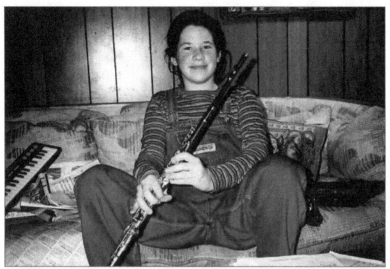

First Musical Instrument She Played. My, how she ministered to us and others with her flute.

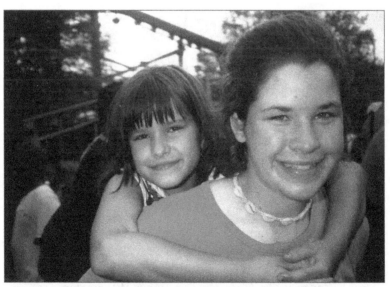

Loved to Carry Laura on Her Shoulders. Laura enjoying a piggy-back ride on her big sister's back.

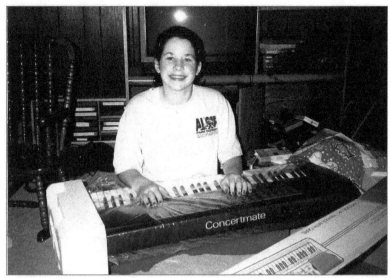

A Perfect Gift She Loved. She loved to play this new keyboard.

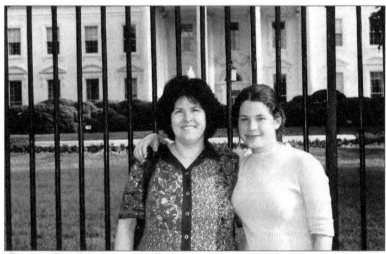

Washington, D.C., 2001. Katie and Pat in front of The White House. Katie qualified for a Spelling Bee in Washington, D.C., in 8th grade.

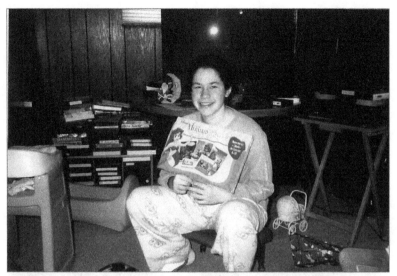

Katie's Favorite Disney Princess. Her favorite Disney character was Ariel from the Little Mermaid.

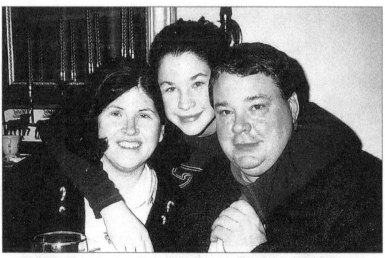

We Will Hug Again! She was always trying to squirm her way between us! Why not, after seeing this photo, give your loved ones a great big hug today.

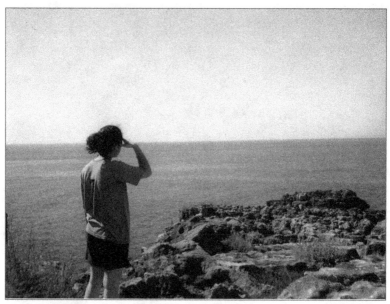

Portugal 2004. Katie gazing over the Atlantic Ocean. This trip truly changed her life.

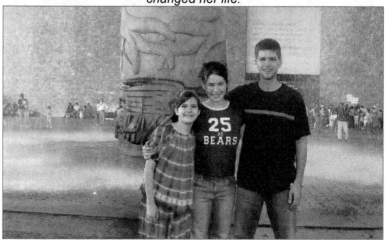

Mexico City 2004. We went to visit Brian when he studied in Mexico for three months.

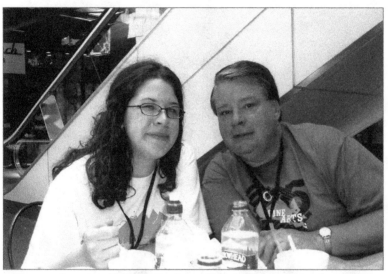

Denver Lunch with Dad. During a little break in the action, Jerry encouraged Katie to get her song "Remembering the Persecuted" recorded by University of Valley Forge, which was offering free recordings. We are so thankful Katie recorded her song, as this song still touches people today.

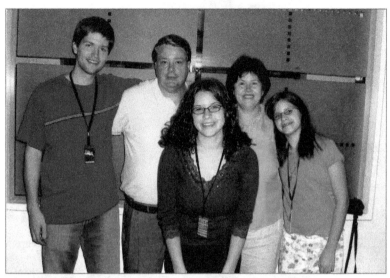

Jerry and Pat's 25th Wedding Anniversary, August 2005, in Denver. Posing for a family photo after Jerry and Pat renewed their wedding vows.

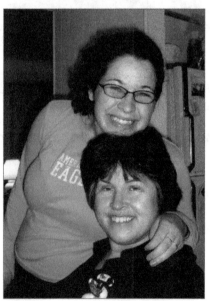

Smiling for a photo with Mom on Christmas.

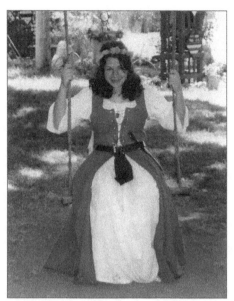

Katie at the Renaissance Faire, which reminds us of what she could be doing in Heaven.

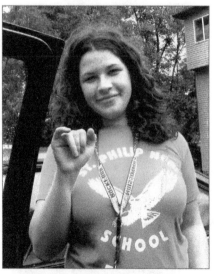

Katie waving goodbye when we dropped her off at the beginning of Rockford Master's Commission.

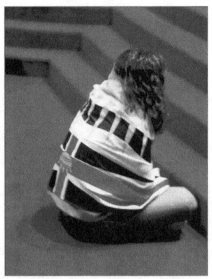

Katie in prayer at Rockford First Church. She wrapped the flags of nations around her as she prayed for her upcoming missions trip to Vancouver. She went to be with the Lord less than a week before her scheduled trip. God truly had other plans.

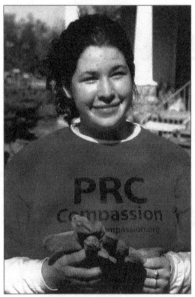

Katie helping with relief work after Hurricane Rita.

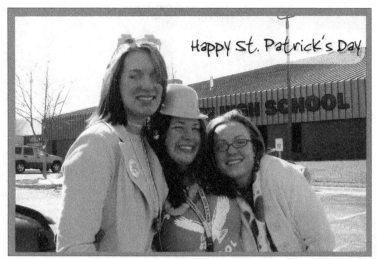

St. Patrick's Day, 2006. The last picture we ever took of Katie. She was with her two friends, Amanda and Christy, from Rockford Master's Commission.

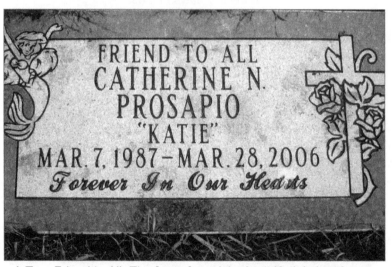

A True Friend to All. The four of us picked out Katie's headstone. We thought it would be fitting to put her favorite princess Ariel on her headstone.

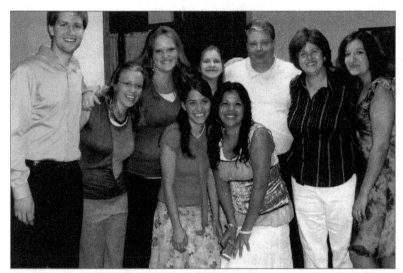

Katie's Scheduled Graduation Day, June 2006. Our family was invited to attend as the lives of Katie and Wendi were honored as part of the ceremony. It was a blessing to be a part of this night with some of Katie's friends.

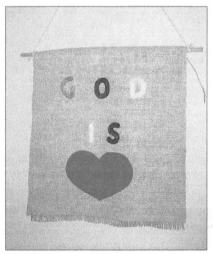

"God is Love" Banner. Katie made this banner when she was six years old. This was one of five items she asked us to bring for her when we visited her the final time.

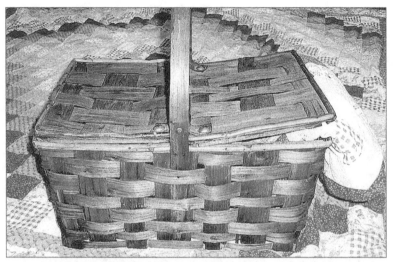

Katie's Picnic Basket. She bought this picnic basket because she very much wanted to have picnics with her friends. This was another one of the items she requested us to bring her on our visit. We bring it wherever the Lord sends us to share the story of Katie's life.

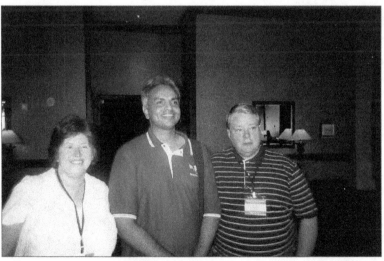

Gospel for Asia Conference. Picture of Pat, Bishop Simon John, and Jerry

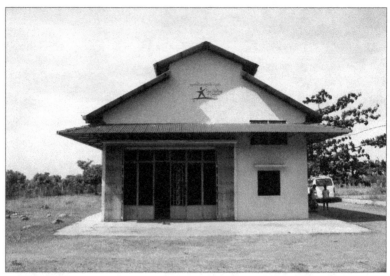

Teen Challenge Center Katie Hall. This first Teen Challenge center in Cambodia is named after Katie. Many lives are being changed daily at this center.

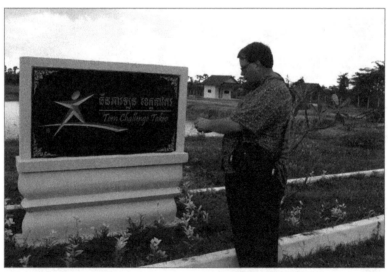

Jerry Scattering Wheat Seeds at Katie Hall. Believing for new life on a previously cursed ground, Jerry scattered wheat seeds from the sheaf of wheat on Katie's casket onto the property of Katie Hall.

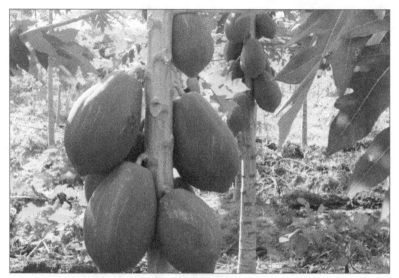

An abundance of crops from the Lord at Katie Hall. The ground is no longer cursed!

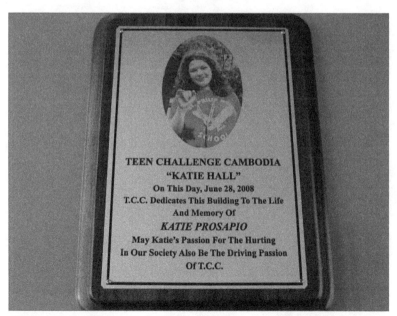

**TEEN CHALLENGE CAMBODIA
"KATIE HALL"**
On This Day, June 28, 2008
T.C.C. Dedicates This Building To The Life
And Memory Of
KATIE PROSAPIO
May Katie's Passion For The Hurting
In Our Society Also Be The Driving Passion
Of T.C.C.

Plaque Hung Inside Katie Hall in Memory of Her Life and Passion.

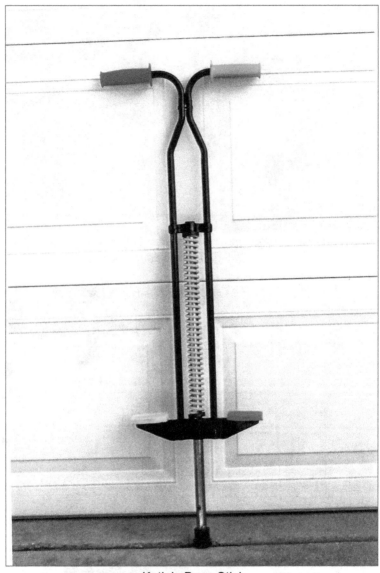

Katie's Pogo Stick

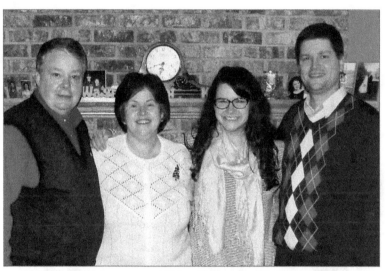

Jerry, Pat, Laura, and Brian Prosapio, Christmas 2014

Chapter Eight

Ready, Set, Go!

(Written by Katie's Dad, Jerry)

"Then I heard the voice of the Lord saying, 'Whom shall I send? And who will go for us?' And I said, 'Here am I. Send me!'" Isaiah 6:8

*P*at and I, as most parents do, try to get special gifts to give our children for Christmas. Earlier in the month, Katie asked Pat and me to consider a different type of gift that we could give her. She shared with us that for the past few months, she was supporting a missionary in India on a $30.00 a month pledge. Her mother and I were not surprised by the country she would want to support, but we were surprised by her being able financially pledge that amount while in the Master's Commission program. She told us that she had fallen behind three months and asked if instead of a Christmas present, we could send a payment to Gospel for Asia for the missionary she was sponsoring.

I was aware of Gospel for Asia, as Katie had given me a book the summer before by its founder, K.P. Yohannan, titled, *Revolution in World Missions*. It is a book that impacted Katie as well as myself upon reading it. One part of the book that Katie had underlined stated, "In some way, which I still do not really understand, the trying of our faith works patience and hope into the fabric of our Christian lives. No one, I am convinced, will follow Jesus very long without tribulation. It is His way of demonstrating His presence. Sufferings and trials—like persecution—are a normal part of the Christian walk. We must learn to accept them, and I think this is true for ministries as well as individuals." It was not at all a difficult decision to send the three-month offering in Katie's name to Gospel for Asia to continue support for her missionary in India. Her mom and I still wanted her to open some presents, so Katie still had some small gifts to open.

After Katie's death, we decided to continue to support Katie's missionary, and we contacted Gospel for Asia to inform them and change the account mailing name from Katie to our name. They had heard about her song "Remembering the Persecuted" and contacted us about an upcoming international conference that they were hosting in Dallas. Hundreds of missionaries from India, as well as supporters from their ministry, would be coming to hear stories and pray for the needs of those missionaries.

They asked Pat and me if we would come to the conference so they could share Katie's story and song with those in attendance. We needed to let them know by the following Monday so they could schedule us into the program. The Sunday before letting them know was my first Father's Day without Katie. It was a very emotional day for me, and although Pat was working, I was blessed to have Brian and Laura with me. I was alone downstairs thinking about what decision needed to be made, when I felt the Lord comfort me. He told me that as an earthly father, there was nothing more I could do with Katie that I had not already done before. She was with Him and everything she was now experiencing was just what she had desired. I began to weep knowing that Katie was with the True Love of her life. I once again realized what a privilege it was to be her father for the nineteen years He had given her to me.

Immediately after my pondering, the phone rang, and I heard the voices of our dear friends from Maryland, Danny and Barbara Peterson. They told me they were in church earlier in the day and were praying for me, knowing this was my first Father's Day without Katie. They then proceeded to share with me that not just one of them, but both of them together, were thinking about Katie and her song. They both heard from the Lord that they were to help in a monetary way to support this song to go out to others. I was once again amazed by the Lord, as they had no idea about the upcoming conference in Dallas.

The amount that the Lord prompted them to give us was the same amount for Pat and me to go to the conference. On the following day, we informed Gospel for Asia that we would be coming, and two weeks later, we arrived at the conference. We met with the program director before it began and asked if he wanted us to come up to the stage or just stand up from our seats when they shared Katie's story and song. We told him we would be more comfortable just standing up in the audience.

The program director decided to share her song before an all-night prayer meeting for needs of missionaries. He displayed a photo of Katie on a large screen and shared about her love and support for her missionary. He then acknowledged that we, her parents, were at the conference but did not have us stand up (that was all right with Pat and me as we were having quite an emotional moment together). They proceeded to play her song and after it ended, there was such a hush and presence of the Holy Spirit that came over the crowd.

The next morning was the final session, and the speaker was a missionary from India named Simon John. He had a powerful and stirring testimony of how he was called out of a successful career to become a missionary. He shared that for three weeks in a row, in different churches, he heard the same Bible story from John 21:15-17, about Simon, son of John, and the Lord telling him to feed His sheep. He became angry after the first Sunday, and he left that church to go 25 miles to another church, but he heard the same message there. Getting more disturbed, he traveled 100 miles the following Sunday to once again hear the same message for him to feed Christ's sheep. He knew then that it was truly the time to surrender and follow the plan God had for Him, to leave behind his job and become a missionary.

The weekend concluded with a communion service. To prepare for it, as there were 2,000 in attendance, the organizers asked everyone to take a fifteen minute break by going into the lobby area. Pat went to the restroom while I waited in the lobby. It was the largest lobby area I had ever seen in a hotel, as we were staying in the expansive Gaylord Hotel. I was standing outside the restroom when a person started coming towards me and our eyes locked with one another. It was Simon John, who had just shared his life story and calling with us. He was heading towards me, and a small voice inside me knew something was about to happen. He came up to me, we extended a handshake to each other, and I thanked him for sharing his life testimony with me. He asked me what it was that brought me to the conference. I began by saying to him, "The song played last night..." and he interrupted me before I could finish my thought. He said, "Was that your daughter who wrote and sang that song?" I said yes. He told me that while it played he wept. He also told me that the Lord Jesus put in his heart that the song was to be played around the world, to encourage others facing persecution for their faith. He then asked me where my wife Pat was, as he wanted to meet her and take a photo of us three to bring back to India. I told him Pat would be back soon, and he waited to meet her and take that photo. Pat shared with me that while she was in the ladies' room, a woman came up to her and asked her if she was the mom of the girl who had sung the song the night before. She told Pat that she and her husband were sitting a row behind us, and she witnessed our emotions as the song was being played. She also told Pat what an impact the words and song meant to her.

From the moment of the invitation, to the financial provision to go to the conference, to the weekend with the most humble, yet giving, missionaries we had time to spend with, we knew that God wanted us to be there. The words of Simon John have come to pass, as Katie's song has and continues to be played at missions and persecuted church conferences around the world.

Six months after Katie's death, I was driving back home after dropping off Laura at school. Less than three blocks from the school, I observed the aftermath of a terrible car accident where two cars had collided. I, along with another motorist, rushed up to the car that was damaged much worse than the other one. Inside, there was a woman who was trapped inside the vehicle, unconscious and bleeding from the crash. We were unable to get her out of the car. I immediately thought to start praying for this woman and was able to reach into the window to touch her shoulder. There was no response, and I could tell that just a little life was left in her body. The other man, when hearing me pray for her, told me to get away from the car. He backed away due to the leaking gas, but I could only keep praying because I knew this was the best thing I could do for her until help arrived.

Minutes later, an elderly man who was the driver of the other car stumbled towards me with a dazed look in his eyes. He was in shock from the accident, and I left the woman's car to help hold him and try to keep him from seeing the lady who he had collided with in the accident. I talked to him and stayed with him until the paramedics came upon the scene and escorted him into an ambulance. I knew there was nothing else I could do and proceeded to get back into my car to drive home. I drove a few blocks and had to pull into a parking lot, as the whole experience of what I had just seen moved me to tears. I realized so clearly that just months before, a team of first responders had been called to come upon the accident of my daughter. I knew God wanted me to witness what these people had to go through.

An article in the next day's newspaper reported that the woman had died in the crash. I told Laura when she came home from school about the woman's death. She immediately asked if I, and her mother Pat, would be going to the wake. I honestly had not even thought of doing that, as it just seemed strange not knowing the woman. Laura then said it might help the family for us to go to pay our respects. Pat and I decided to go. When we got to the front by the casket, we met the woman's only daughter. I explained to her that I had come upon the accident scene and was there to pray for her mom. I also shared that she did not suffer and that when I came up to the car she was unconscious and not in any pain.

Upon telling her this, she broke out in tears and thanked and hugged me. She said that the question she had unanswered was whether or not her precious mother had suffered. She proceeded to introduce us to other relatives so I could share that with them. Pat was also able to minister to the family by sharing about Katie's recent death and knowing what this family was going through due to such a sudden loss. When Pat and I left the funeral home, we sat a while in the car, sensing God's timing in all of what occurred between two grieving families.

It was shortly after this that I was driving once again and did something I had never done before. I spoke out verbally, "God, I am ready." I was startled as I was not in the habit of audibly talking to God by myself, let alone while driving the car. Hearing the words I had said and feeling they were well meant left me shaken and a bit afraid. I then said, "God, Pat and I are ready." We had recently talked about being open to going where the Lord wanted us so that we could share our journey with others.

Pat was in the house when I arrived home, and I told her about what had happened in the car and how I first said "God, I am ready" and then how I included her in my declaration to God. She was surprised by how it happened, as she knew I do not speak out like that, let alone to God while driving the car. Minutes later, we heard the mailman come by, and we went to retrieve our daily mail in the box. There was a letter addressed to us from Trinity Christian College. It was written by a counselor who was teaching a course on grief and loss. She asked if we would be able to come and share our story with her class. She had heard about Katie and her song, "Remembering the Persecuted," and she listened to it quite often. She was always moved to tears by the prayer and passion within Katie's words. "She said that to ask to have faith like the persecuted church is what the essence of this class will be dealing with. Can we in the face of heartache and hardship trust in a loving God?" After reading the letter and the invitation to share with the students, Pat and I just sat motionless for awhile. **Does God work that soon after you say you are ready?** We both agreed it was Him that was opening the door for us to share our journey with this class and counselor. We sent the response back with a couple dates, with one of them falling on Pat's birthday, January 22nd.

We assembled packets of a few of Katie's writings, as well as a CD of her songs to give to each of the students. It seemed right to stack them into one of Katie's special possessions: a picnic basket that Katie had bought from a local thrift store. It was an item that Katie had asked us to bring on our last visit to her in Rockford, ten days before she went to be with the Lord. I remember packing it in the trunk of the car on a rather cold March day and saying to myself, "Why does she want this picnic basket?" When we arrived in Rockford and unpacked the car, I asked Katie that question, and her answer was that she wanted to have a picnic with her friends. I was happy to see Katie, and even though her wanting to have a picnic in the cold did not make sense to me, I handed her the picnic basket to bring up to her room.

When Katie's possessions came back to us after her death, we stored them downstairs in a room until it was the right time to go through them. Pat found a journal of Katie's in which she wrote a beautiful letter to God about Heaven. It contained so many metaphors that Katie, in her childlike yet immense love for God, wrote. Pat, with tears in her eyes, showed me this "Heaven letter." I too got teary eyed when I read through to the end of the letter. Her last sentence was, "Let's go for a picnic." It immediately made me think of her picnic basket, and I gazed across the room to see Katie's basket seemingly staring back at me. I sensed there was a definite connection about what we were to do in the future with this basket. We have since had many picnics with family and friends, with our food packed away in the picnic basket. We have always brought Katie's letter about Heaven with us on picnics to share with others.

When we exited our car on that snowy, wintry day (which was Pat's birthday) at Trinity Christian College, it seemed strange to others, but just right to us, to walk through the campus with a picnic basket to speak to a class on grief and loss. In the class, we shared Katie's life and writings, and the counselor played one of her songs to end the class. It was a very emotional day for all of us, but as the counselor closed the class, she mentioned, "There are singers in this room who have yet to write their own song to God." Before the students left class, they surprised us by singing "Happy Birthday" to Pat. We were so blessed to be able to speak to these students and to share our loss, but more importantly, to share our hope of seeing our precious Katie again and having that picnic in Heaven with her and so many other loved ones.

Chapter Nine

Continuing Onward

(Written by the Prosapio Family)

"However, I consider my life worth nothing to me; my only aim is to finish the race and complete the task the Lord Jesus has given me—the task of testifying to the good news of God's grace." Acts 20:24

Katie's passing continues to touch and lead our lives in various ways. Following are just a few examples of how each of us honors the memory of Katie in our everyday lives.

Pat

It is an honor to be called "Mom" and to be a part of raising precious gifts from God. Nine years after Katie's passing, I continue to minister to other moms who have lost children, as well as minister to other needs the Lord places on my heart, such as individuals who have experienced the death of spouse or are suffering from a serious illness.

Whenever I hear of a loss of a child, my heart is so grieved. I never would have had this level of compassion had I not gone through the death of my own daughter. I want to reach out to help that mom whose world is suddenly shattered. I want to ease her deep pain of loss, the feeling that part of one's heart and soul has been ripped out. I want to offer hope that someday she will laugh again and have joy at the gifts God has given her.

I realize that with the loss of a child, a mom could easily escape into a deep depression and be angry at God and not want to be part of life in the present. It is a choice to make. I choose life, and I know Katie would want me to. I am thankful for all of the gifts God gives us each day. For example, I love watching Brian and Laura grow into a deeper relationship with Jesus and watch their level of trust in Him.

When I reach out to a grieving mom by giving her a comfort basket, I find I am touching her heart and letting her know that I understand and care about her and what has just happened. I then ask her to tell me about her child and what he or she was like. It is so important to talk about her child and say the child's precious name; it is like music to the grieving mom's ears. We will never tire of hearing their names. So often, well-meaning family and friends feel it will hurt the grieving mom if they "bring up her child's name." What they don't understand is that child is already in their thoughts and minds each day.

If there is one thing I would like to share with others, it is to remember the birthday and anniversary of death day of the loved one and reach out with a phone call or card, just to let them know that you care. We have the most wonderful family and friends who walk alongside us on our grief journey. One family gives us a beautiful bouquet of yellow roses (Katie's favorite) each anniversary of Katie's passing. It is like a balm for our souls and makes our family so thankful that someone remembers our precious child's life.

In Katie's final letter to me, she told me that as I reach out to others, God would give me more and more love to give to others. She then wrote, "It's really cool how God works, isn't it?" It truly is, Katie! I want to leave a legacy like you did. Thank you for showing me the way to give to others. Until we meet again! What a reunion it will be!

Brian

As my sister Laura mentioned in an earlier chapter, one of the last conversations that our family had with Katie centered on the topic of grace. Grace can be described with the acrostic, "God's Riches At Christ's Expense." It is receiving all of God's blessings for us, because Jesus paid the punishment for our sins on the cross. The greatest blessing that we receive is the gift of eternal life with Jesus in Heaven. This is a free gift for us, if we choose to believe on Jesus and accept this gift. As the Scriptures say in Ephesians 2:8-10, "For it is by grace you have been saved, through faith—and this not from yourselves, it is the gift of God—not by works, so that no one can boast. For we are God's workman-ship, created in Christ Jesus to do good works, which God prepared in advance for us to do." As this Scripture says, grace cannot be earned or deserved by our good works. However, our good works flow out of gratitude for receiving this new life in Christ Jesus.

Yet, the Scriptures also show it is possible to forget about the concept of grace and to start living as if one still needs to earn his or her way to God. As the apostle Paul wrote to the church in Galatia, "I do not set aside the grace of God, for if righteousness could be gained through the law, Christ died for nothing (Galatians 2:21)!" I can relate to this passage, because there was a period in my life when I had set aside the grace of God, thinking that I had to do certain things to remain in God's favor. I had forgotten that God's grace had already covered all of my mistakes and shortcomings that I thought were keeping me from God.

Paul went on to tell the Galatians, "I have been crucified with Christ and I no longer live, but Christ lives in me. The life I live in the body, I live by faith in the Son of God, who loved me and gave himself for me (Galatians 2:20)." As I heard someone once say, it is a good thing to live the dead life. No, not as a zombie, which is common in popular culture, but as someone who is dead to sin and alive in Christ. As Paul told the Galatians, "Those who belong to Christ Jesus have crucified the sinful nature with its passions and desires. Since we live by the Spirit, let us keep in step with the Spirit (Galatians 5:24-25)." Moreover, Paul told the Galatians, "So I say, live by the Spirit, and you will not gratify the desires of the sinful nature." As we accept God's grace in our life, His Spirit will help us live the life He desires for us.

The concept of grace is something I have taken to heart the past several years. My sister Katie helped to plant this seed in my life, and it is something that I keep returning to as I walk down the path of life. I think, in some ways, we naturally try to resist the idea of grace, because we live in a society that seems to value hard work and performance above all else. Yet, as we see in these biblical passages, the gift of eternal life is something we cannot earn or deserve. It is something that we accept as a gift and give thanks to God for.

.I continually thank God for saving me by His grace, and I thank Him for using my sister Katie to teach me the importance of grace. Nine years have passed since my sister's homegoing to Heaven, but I know she is up there encouraging each one of us, along with the great cloud of witnesses gone before us, to continue to "Grow in the grace and knowledge of our Lord and Savior Jesus Christ. To Him be glory both now and forever! Amen (2 Peter 3:18)."

Laura

Just the week after Katie passed away, I had to express my emotions in some way. There was so much chaos happening around me and in me that I needed to put what I was feeling down on paper. This habit of expressing my feelings of grief has continued throughout the last nine years, and I'm thankful that I can look back and read how my feelings have changed as time has gone by. I'd like to share a few these poems with you so that you can witness my journey through the grief of losing someone I love so dearly. As you read, I encourage you to note the hopelessness in the beginning of my journey contrasted by the sense of comfort that accompanies the later poems.

"Bittersweet"—Age 12

Distressed yet uplifted,
Confusing yet clear,
She's up there but she's still here.
Making new memories...what are memories anymore?
Seems like the beginning, but is it the end?
One second back, one minute forward
Would life still be an option?
Did she hurt? Was there pain?
Well, I feel pain.
I don't see the purpose, but it's staring right at me.
Can this whole thing be?
Is this a dream?
One week before, holding her hand.
Her hand under the ground.
Worthless are those thoughts.
Don't think that way!
That laugh, that smile, that hug.
Long will it be for that, but short?
Understanding...seems overrated.
Just a stop in my life.
A turning point.
So sudden it seems.

"Year's Past Emotions"—Age 13

I had a sudden rush of feelings
Like the accident just happened,
A temporary lapse of reason.
It felt like nobody understood,
And that she'd be walking home tonight
To the place she's always known as home
And the girl who always was known as her sister.
But it's not that way,
It'll never be.
No matter how much I try
This earthly home will never be enough.
Heaven is sufficient
For the longing that I feel,
That promise I hold dear.
Yet it still seems like forever
Until the day she runs down that golden street,
Until I embrace her,
Until the day when I look into her face.
But now, I am on the waiting list.
How relieved will I feel
When I am taken off hold.
But until then
I am happy to be in this world,
Holding on to memories
That will never be forgotten.

I am not living in the past or in the future,
But the present is where
I am assigned to be.

"Time Goes On But Love Remains"—Age 16

Sometimes I miss you beyond words,
Other times I simply cry.
But most days now are like the rest—
They miraculously go by.

That's not to say I don't care anymore,
For my being aches with love.
But somehow joy has come to stay—
Grief I know less of.

Your hugs impressed upon my shoulders—
The feeling of your hands
Your angelic smile and your ocean blue eyes,
Those soft and curly brown hair strands.

The lovely sound of your voice
That calmed me on the darkest of nights.
The truth that poured out from your lips
Has brought my understanding to new heights.

Memories are quiet and stillborn.
They are hidden deep within,
Yet when I think of my past with you,
I can't help but laugh and grin.

For these memories are different—
Although they are gone and done.
Life springs from my mind with these;
I hear laughs, feel joy, remember fun.

I taste chocolate chip cookie dough ice cream.
I feel the concrete curb underneath.
I peer into the amusing thoughts in your head—
Another smile forms with your teeth.

How I love to recollect
All the joys you've made me feel—
The advice you gave, the love you shared,
The broken hearts you would heal.

I see your name engraved in stone—
"Friend to All" it reads below.
I laugh inside, a tear down my cheek
For a few cherished things I know.

This special person is my sister—
And I was blessed to admire
My hero, my love, my friend, my Katie
Her example to aspire.

While some of the memories have faded—and also a lot of the pain—my love for Katie has not. I find that the tears are becoming more infrequent, and in their place, a smile often surfaces. Katie's life was a part of my life, and even though she is gone from this earth, a part of me still carries Katie's life as a part of me. Now that I'm twenty-one years old, I realize that I have begun to live days that my older sister never got to live. Yet, in the times where I may feel guilty or undeserving of living beyond what she got to live, I realize in my heart that she out of anybody would want me to live everyday filled with abundant joy and happiness. I am developing my own story each day, and I am beyond thankful that Katie's life was able to have a part in my life. I am thankful for the beauty of our memories together and also for the innumerable lessons learned throughout the past nine years of her absence.

I continue to come back to the truth of God's faithfulness in my life. He truly has taken an experience that was not at all easy to walk through, and He has infused purpose into it. He has worked all things together for good (Romans 8:28). I am confident that in the days to come, He will continue to soothe my heart with His comfort whenever I feel grief. When I was so surrounded with death of my sister at such an early age, He gave me the promise of being able to live life abundantly—not only to carry my sister's testimony, but also to live out my own.

For this, I am entirely grateful. God is good all the time, and all the time, God is good.

Jerry

It was at Katie's wake that I found myself saying over and over again to those who came that evening that I was thankful to have been her dad for the nineteen years the Lord had given me. I know that was not anything I planned to say, but when I spoke those words to those who came, I know it truly was with a heart of gratitude. A few weeks after the funeral around 2:00 AM, I woke up and was unable to go back to sleep. I sat in a recliner in our family's living room, and a dark, deep emotion of grief swept over me. It was so powerful and consuming that it brought me to a level of hopelessness that I had never experienced in my life. I prayed for it to leave, but it was so dark with the thoughts of the loss of Katie that I was unable to even get up from the chair. I remember thinking that if this was how future days were going to be, I didn't think I could make it. This experience happened to me on one more occasion, and shortly after these experiences, some of our good friends stopped by to share a video with us about a pastor who had lost his daughter. In the video, the pastor shared that Isaiah 53:3-4 demonstrates how Jesus is acquainted with grief and he has carried our grief. He also shared about how God the Father knows what it is like to have given His only Son to be put to death.

When I watched and heard this Scripture and felt the love of the Father after my losing a child, the impact was life-changing. There would be no more dark, hopeless nights, and if any such thoughts came, I offered them to the Lord, realizing that He alone could bear my grief.

The Lord has planned divine appointment ministry opportunities that He alone could orchestrate. Pat and I were asked by the associate pastor of our church to lead the Sunday evening service, as our senior pastor was not present that day. We agreed to lead the service. That afternoon, Pat reminded me of a video we had recently seen about a pastor who had shared his testimony about a near-death experience. She felt it would be good to bring to church to show to those who came that evening. Much to our surprise, there were only four people in attendance—Pat and I, our sound technician, and a single woman. We waited ten minutes past the start time to begin, but it was still only the four of us. Nevertheless, Pat and I decided to start the video.

When the video ended, the four of us sat in the front two pews to talk. The woman opened her heart to us and shared about her recent struggles with depression. She admitted that earlier that morning, she was unable to get dressed to come to church. She shared how in previous months, she had frequent thoughts of suicide and had even asked God to take her life. She also shared that she was currently on an anti-depressant medication, but that she also wanted to stop taking it in the future.

Pat and I looked into each other's eyes and knew what we needed to share with this woman. It was the right time and the right place to share about Katie and her battle with and victory over depression.

Pat shared with the woman at church about Katie's suicide letter that turned our world upside down. Katie wanted, much like this woman who we were talking with, not to live anymore. As we continued explaining Katie's story, we found that God was comforting her through Katie's testimony.

After sharing Katie's testimony with this lady suffering from depression, the four of us at church that Sunday night ended in prayer for her to be set free from depression in her life. I believe this freedom is available to anyone who, like Katie and this woman we met, is able to **CRY OUT FOR HELP**. One phone call to someone who cares for you can make all the difference! And as the Scriptures say in Romans 10:13, "Everyone who calls on the name of the Lord will be saved."

One day, I picked up my wife Pat after work. She had worked two hours longer than usual due to an admission of a baby at the hospital where she is employed. She had not been able to have a lunch that day due to other emergency situations, so she was really hungry for dinner.

I suggested we eat out, and I gave her a choice of two restaurants.

We went to the restaurant she picked out and had a great meal served by a wonderful waitress. She was in her mid-twenties and had a special warmness that both Pat and I noticed and commented on after finishing our dinner.

When the check came, I asked Pat if she had a Katie's Comfort Ministry card on her, which we sometimes leave with our tip. Pat had one on her, and we left it with the tip on the table. Pat needed to use the restroom, so I waited by the exit door in front of the restaurant for her.

I was looking out the door with my back to the restroom when I heard a voice from behind me trying to get my attention. I turned to see our waitress holding the ministry card in her hand. She asked me, "Were you Katie's Dad?" I was a bit startled, but my answer came out, "Yes, I am."

She then said she knew Katie, as they were both on the speech team together in high school. With tears forming in her eyes, she told me she is the person she is today because of Katie. Katie encouraged her at a time in her life when she needed it the most, and Katie let her know that God loved her. Katie would also pray with her and because of the love Katie showed her, she is still following God today.

Trying to get my emotions in check, I asked her what her name was, and she told me it was Angie. I then told her that my wife Pat was in the restroom. Angie proceeded to meet Pat there and share the same story that she just shared with me. When Pat asked her what her name was and found out that it was Angie, Pat remembered that Katie had written about Angie in the margin of a book she was reading during her studies at Rockford Master's Commission. Katie had written her name in her *Purpose Driven Life* book, with a note to pray for Angie and to give her a phone call. When Pat shared this with Angie, it made her tear up even more. Yet, Angie was crying tears of happiness because she realized that Katie had been praying and thinking about her.

Pat and I believe only God could have led us to this restaurant seven years later to meet a beautiful young woman named Angie, someone whose life was changed through meeting our precious daughter Katie. May each of us be similarly used by God to reach out to those around us in need.

Chapter Ten

From Darkness to Light

(Katie's Journal Writings)

"Therefore, I urge you, brothers and sisters, in view of God's mercy, to offer your bodies as a living sacrifice, holy and pleasing to God—this is your true and proper worship. Do not conform to the pattern of this world, but be transformed by the renewing of your mind. Then you will be able to test and approve what God's will is—his good, pleasing and perfect will." Romans 12:1-2

To share how God brought Katie out of depression, we thought it best to share some of her journal writings with you. These writings span from the early depths

of her struggle with depression to her final writings a
month before going to be with Jesus in Heaven.

Poems of Depression

Everyone who passed by her
Lifeless soul
Thought that some presence
Still breathed beneath her eyes.

Nothing could tear her
From enigmatic feeling
She was only detached
From her own darkness.

I am falling
The world is caving in
So much to deal with
But I can't anymore
I just can't
I've waited for long empty nights
For a sign that someone cares about me
That a random being would reach out
But no one has
No one could reach out to someone like me
Because I am ugly, fat, and stupid

And no one cares
I feel like everyone is watching me
Pointing and laughing every time I turn around
I am completely naïve to the people around me.

Balance, tipping
Trying to hide
I want to draw my blood
Watch it flow down slowly
Become numb again

I am disconnected
A roaming child,
Lost, waiting for someone
To find me in this solitude

Hope is my only friend
Even though it betrays me
I am drained of life
Still worse I am becoming

Blood flows from my lips
My eyes are charred and hard
I feel like a man doomed to die
There is no time left

The walls around me block my vision
Tears spring to my eyes
Where is the hope I used to feel?
Why is it hiding in the depths of my soul?
Where I can't tell if it's even there

I am separated
Once I was collected
My thoughts were one,
Now I don't know
What to think or what
to feel anymore

Why can't I open up my eyes
Why can't I run through the rivers of my soul
I feel like a part of my soul has died
And my heart will never again be whole

I can't live like this
Slipping off the edge of uncertainty
I feel like I don't even exist
I am just passing through a road
And the only reason I know I am
alive is my shadow,
which contains more life
Than my mind and soul

"Secret"

Do you want to hear a secret?
It might change your heart
It might bring us together
Or drive us apart

Here goes nothing
I hate myself
I hate my cries
I hate the world
I hate the lies.

I want to
Make you see
I'm not okay
And I'll never be

You're so pure and innocent
I don't want you to think like me
But you must know the truth
How I'll never be free

I hate myself
I hate my cries
I hate the world
I hate the lies

I want to
Make you see
I'm not okay
And I'll never be

I feel like I'm hidden
I'm always wearing a mask
I just want you to know
Is that too much to ask?

"The Realm of My Past"

Wondering about nothing and everything
My mind drifts to the forgotten ruins
Of my former and happier life—
Childhood

I used to play in the sand
And race to be the first one on the swings
I used to laugh at everything,
Not knowing what was pain

When did life become so complicated?
Did the earth fall upside-down?
I hope that one day I can truly live again
But I am afraid I will never be free

Wondering about nothing and everything
My mind drifts to the forgotten ruins
Of my former and happier life—
Childhood

"My Eulogy"

On this Christmas Eve,
I want to die.
No one but me knows why.

My mind has been broken
My heart has been crushed
I can no longer go on.

I sacrificed everything for you
But you didn't even realize it
You just stared.

I gave everything to you
But you continue to demand
More than I could ever give

All of my dreams are gone
All my hopes are shattered
All I have left is empty thoughts.

On this Christmas Eve,
I want to die.
No one but me knows why.

Poems and Writings about Victory over Depression

"Testimony"

I knew Jesus since I was a child, but then I started living for myself and others instead of Him. I became very depressed. I would want to sit at home by myself and would always feel like there was a cloud around me. It was very hard because I felt like there was no hope. When people asked me what I wanted to do when I graduated high school, I did not know what to say because I could not see anything but a black hole. It was hard for me to go to school because all I wanted to do was sleep, and I did not find anything I had used to find interesting worth doing anymore. It was a really hard time, but after I went on a missions trip to Portugal and saw that God was at work in different parts of the world, I knew that He wanted to help me, too. So, I gave my life to Him. Now, I have hope.

"Portugal"

The first rays of dawn shine through the window pane,
All is silent but the birds' cheerful song.

Which seems to travel on the breeze as it makes its way to my ear.

Soon the town will be bustling with shop talk and cheerful greetings.

I can almost see the children greet each other with a kiss to either side of the cheek.

An image that is cliché, yet filled with truth and compassion.

The sight brings warmth to my heart, a comfort that reassures the love of this place.

In some ways, it feels like home, like I've lived here my entire life.

The weary sun begins to set, as another day in this picturesque world diminishes into history.

With child-like enthusiasm, I await tomorrow's coming, and the new wonders and miracles it brings with it.

Along with a joy that comes only to those who seek it.

Blank faces
That stare at me
Asking me why I
am so happy

I smile and tell them
That life is more than
a week of days,
more than a person in the
world.

It's a chance to be reborn,
A chance to be made new.

But they do not understand
the joy I feel
The overwhelming feeling that
my life will change another's
heart.
That my tears are not in vain,
That my smile can brighten
someone's day.

They wait for me to get angry
at them or at the world
for its horrible wickedness,
but I look beyond the evil
and see the good,
because light always overcomes all darkness.

Wasted away
It's time to shine
You don't have
To struggle anymore
When the world tries to unite
Itself on your heart
God smiles and says,

She's mine.

Don't hurt
You have nothing to lose but your life
Sometime years from now
You'll know how God calmed you
How he's so close sometimes
You can't even recognize Him.

Pressed down
Like foreign flowers
Between pages of indecision
Somewhere there has to be an answer.
Tomorrow I want to love you
But all I have is today
And if I'm really gonna do your will
Then I guess that means giving you everything
All the dreams I ever had for myself
Every hope
It is yours.

I can move my fingers and wiggle my toes.
I can open my eyes to the beautiful world.

I have such a life to live
That will only be lived once.

I want to make a difference in this world
And live every moment of life joyfully and expectantly.

Not everyone will like me, my smile may not be
returned by all
But it only takes one person to spur a change.

I am not promised tomorrow, only today
So with every last breath in my body
I gaze up into the stars wondering what will happen in
the future.

I am only a citizen of my own respite
And resistant of my own pursuit.

I may feel alone
But I will always have a guardian.

The following writings were found in Katie's RMC Journals. They were written about one month before she went to be with the Lord.

God, you mean so much to me. You gripped me from the jaws of death and saved me. You have held me in your arms and touched me in miraculous ways. Through everything, friends coming and going, change of environments, emotions, everything, You have been faithful. I thank you for letting me experience pain so I could fully understand the hurt of your people. You have brought me from the pit of disillusionment and depression. You are amazing and clever and creative. You fill all of the empty spaces of my heart, making me whole inside and out. You are my friend through everything and you won't abandon me no matter what.

Worship is giving all you have to God, not just in song but in your life. It means making everything you do be an extension of pure, deep love and awe of God. In the form of song, it is telling God how much He means to you, how much you love Him. It's pausing for moments to revere Him and treat Him like who He is. In a worship service, giving to God is more important than receiving from Him. It's not about us or the goosebumps or feeling ministered to, though these things may occur. It's to touch His heart, not ours. As the song says, "It's all about you, Jesus."

It's moments like these where I know that I've grown up. I'm not the same person I was when I came here. I am not insecure anymore. I am not scared. I am not shy.

I'm not afraid of other people anymore or of what they think. I'm not afraid to think, learn, grow, to change.

Before, I had just assumed or got comfortable thinking I knew just enough. I knew that if I didn't know, I wouldn't have to move or stretch.

I prayed for God to invade my comfort zones, but I didn't really mean it. When He would tell me to do something especially hard, I was terrified! But I know it was right. I'm not afraid of branching out or stepping off. I'm not afraid to say no. I know now that I don't have to do things for people to get them to like me. It's not my responsibility to be likable. It is my responsibility to be whom God has made me to be—<u>without apology</u>.

Thank you, Lord, that I can make mistakes and that's o.k. I learned that insecurity can be deadly and how important it is to speak the truth without being afraid of how it is taken. Because the truth will set people free, even if it hurts their feelings. My job on this earth is <u>not</u> to make people like me or approve of me. How hollow is that. It's something I could never attain, even if I tried for my whole life. People are not my god. You are, and I worship You, and I exalt You above my feelings and give no room in my heart for fear that does not come from You. I worship You in absolute surrender and abandonment, Lord. I want to <u>know</u> Your voice.

God, I refuse to get comfortable. I dare to move. Even when I go back home, I resolve to push and fight for my freedom, for my time spent with You, for the convictions

You've placed within my spirit, for the words You've hand-written on my heart.

I will not settle, because if I do, I will fall down like Alka-Seltzer or wine sediment. No, I will fight. I will move. I will fail. I will fight. I will get right back up. I will push. I will not wait. I will stand, and after I have done all, I will still stand.

I will live in God. I will not quit or back down just because it's hard. God, I pray that even now you would give me the fortitude for when I go back home, yet the desire to gain and be and move all I can here, and to reach past every limitation I thought I had.

God, I thank you that I am not a slave to fear. Instead, I have received the spirit of sonship, by which I cry, "Daddy, Father."

It is Valentine's Day, 2006, and I love you, God. I have never had a happier Valentine's Day in my entire life. I'm so content just to be with You. I need/<u>want</u> nothing else.

Something special
something beautiful
original
you've placed in me
i am

not anyone else
just me

spectacular
a shooting star
someone who soars
above everything
free from everything
that once constrained me
i am ready
to change the world today

i am unknown
yet whispered upon
i am one, yet many
i am alone, yet surrounded
together, yet apart
something rescinded, yet kept
something you've placed your hand on
my heart

Things I wanna do:

1. Write an influential book that makes people think and see things in a new way.

2. Play a guitar and sing in a coffee shop dimly lit with a curtain and stage.

3. Act out with all my soul and sing in a musical. Be the character. Do it. Don't be afraid.

4. Write the best song ever.

5. Ride a horse into open fields.
6. Skydive.

This is the final entry that we found in Katie's journal, written three days before she went to be with the Lord.

Find me here
Rain on me
Refresh my soul with your waters
Until I'm changed forever
I want to be with you
right now, you are all I seek
And I've come here
Because I need a touch from you
Because another day without you is impossible to bear
Because I can stand strong on you
When nothing else in my life makes sense

I'm right before you, God
naked and exposed
You see everything in me
There is nothing I can hide
Because you know every secret
That's passed from my breath
Because you know every hair
That is on my head

Because you listen for me
In the quiet watches of the night
Because you long for me greater
Than I could ever long for you

Because when you see me,
Your heart burns for me
Because you long to be with me
As I long to be with you
Because you love me so deeply and fiercely
Even when I've turned away from it
How often have I resisted you

Because when I sin
It breaks your heart
Because your love never changes
Even when my love does
Because your love is better than life
And it is everywhere
Because even when I can't feel you
You are with me
Because your face is the first thing I want to see
every morning
Because you are good, the deepest kind
Like marshmallows crackling on a fire
Like a new puppy that just came home to a little kid
Like a grill to George Foreman

Like a word after 40 years of silence
Like a symphony as its beauty is being integrated

On a Sunday afternoon, two days before Katie and Wendi went to be with the Lord, a classmate looked outside her window to capture a joyous moment she would later share with our family. She saw Katie, with her naturally curly hair, jumping up and down on her pogo stick. This pogo stick was one of the items Katie had asked us to bring to her when we came to visit her ten days prior. This classmate shared how happy Katie looked and how only Katie, at age 19, could have the joy she had with her pogo stick! We believe Katie is still jumping for joy in Heaven with her one true love, Jesus. We journey each day missing Katie on this side of Heaven; but instead of dwelling on what we have lost, we continue to remember what Katie has gained!

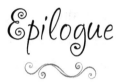

Epilogue

*I*t has now been nine years since Katie's death; yet, at times, she seems more alive than ever. A ministry aptly named, "Katie's Comfort Ministry," was birthed in 2008. It is a family effort by all four of us, with the prayers and support of so many who knew and loved Katie. Our mission statement is: **To bring God's hope and healing to grieving and hurting families, to minister to people who are suffering from depression, and to bring awareness to others to pray for Christians in persecuted areas around the world.**

Pat continues to attend a local monthly grief support group for mothers who have lost children. She has found purpose in reaching out to new mothers who come to the group. She also assembles "comfort baskets" for grieving mothers. In these baskets, she includes a tea cup and saucer, a daily reflections book, a picture frame, small stuffed animals, and some edible goodies. Upon hearing about a mother who has lost a child, either by word of mouth, by phone (708-389-1127), or by e-mail (pat@katiescomfort.org), Pat personally delivers a comfort basket or sends it to the mother through the mail. Pat has transformed what was once Katie's bedroom into a ministry room full of baskets, tea cups, and supplies for the next mother in need of comfort.

Laura was also greatly helped by attending a children's grief support group the year after Katie's death. She is now regularly asked by grief organizations to speak at various functions to provide hope for individuals who are grieving. Laura has also reached out to fellow high school and college students who have suffered a loss. She is now a senior in college at Evangel University, studying Psychology and English. She currently volunteers as a group facilitator for teenagers at a grief center near her university called Lost & Found. Additionally, she has helped with editing this book. She is excited for God to use her compassionate heart for people and her writing to bring Him glory. Currently, she is working on a writing project with the focus of helping other individuals who have experienced the loss of a sibling.

Brian continues to help the ministry by maintaining the website, composing e-mail messages, and editing this book. His unselfish attitude and willingness to help the ministry in any way is a tremendous blessing. Brian accompanied Laura to Moody Church in Chicago for a

Conference on the Persecuted Church in 2011. Laura gave an introduction to Katie's song, "Remembering the Persecuted," before it was played to all who were in attendance. It was played during a time of prayer for those who are serving God in persecuted areas of the world.

Jerry continues to answer the day-to-day phone calls to the ministry. He also keeps in contact with those involved with "Katie Hall" in Cambodia, a center that was opened in 2008 by Katie's former children's pastor and his wife, who do missionary work in Southeast Asia. "Katie Hall" is a Teen Challenge Center for young men who live on the streets, are addicted to alcohol and drugs, and have no other place to live. Here, these young men learn about Jesus and how He can change their lives and give them freedom from their addictions. These young men also learn life and occupational skills that they can take with them when they are ready to leave the center. Following is a testimonial from a student who recently graduated from Katie Hall: "At the Teen Challenge Center, they counseled me, taught me various skills, and helped me to realize the dangerous path I was walking down, helped me to start taking responsibility for my life, and find a good pathway to becoming a constructive member of society. They introduced me to God, and it is God who changed me." This is just one of many whose lives have been changed at Katie Hall. It is with great joy to announce that a second center for women and their children opened In 2012. It has become a safe haven to minister to those women and children who need a touch from God on their lives.

Our family continues to to be invited to churches and grief support groups to share our story of hope and God's comfort to others. Jerry and Pat have led a support group series to help others through their journey of grief. Jerry, along with his friend, Ken Darnell, is also involved in a ministry called Gambling Exposed. Ken shares biblical truths about gambling, as well as the negative impact that gambling has had on individuals and communities in this nation. Jerry shares his personal testimony of gambling addiction and how he found freedom from it. Jerry and Ken are available to share their message to youth groups, churches, and other civic organizations upon request. Their website is **www.gamblingexposed.org** .

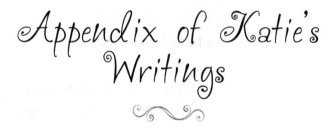

Appendix of Katie's Writings

Song Lyrics

"Remembering the Persecuted"
(Recorded by Katie at the University of Valley Forge recording studio at a National Fine Arts Festival in Denver, Colorado, in August 2005)

God sees everything you do
And you're not fighting this battle alone
Each day hope He spreads anew
He brings joy along with pain
And your sufferings are not in vain
So we'll keep you in our prayers
And know that Jesus cried blood mixed with tears
For the persecuted church
This song goes out to you

Light a candle in the wind
Burn with passion for our King
Love Him like you've always known how
And keep up the faith
We're here behind you

Starving, knocking on secret doors to pray
Hiding places, impressions that will never fade
Blood, sweat, and tears, imprisoned for years
Seeing loved ones die
Right before your eyes

So this song goes out to every secret church
You'll never renounce His Name
Dear God, make my faith like the persecuted church
Bring peace to every cry in silence
Every wound by a gunman share a crown
God, one day I know that I'll be the persecuted church
May I never renounce your Name
May I never be ashamed

Light a candle in the wind
Burn with passion for our King
Love Him like you've always known how
And keep up the faith
We're here behind you now

"I Am Changed"
(Recorded by Katie at Rockford Master's Commission in February 2006)

And all of my longings turn for you.

The sky is white and everything is calm.

And every prayer I whisper reaches straight to
your heart.

And my song is like a million different symphonies in
your soul.

And I am changed by being where the angels walked.

Singing holy is your name, holy is your name.

And I believe that you are as real as the wind,

That brushes up against my heart,

And I know that your gaze is on me,

And you are smiling.

And right now in this moment,

With the trees as my witness,

I choose to give up my life to find yours.

Catches my breath is a passion for you,

Is like a torrent that can't be held back.

The words you speak electrify my senses,

Vibrate in my ears, and capture all consciousness.

And I am changed by being where the angels walked.

Singing holy is your name, holy is your name.

And I believe you are as real as the wind,

That brushes up against my heart,

And I know that your gaze is on me,

And you are smiling.
And right now in this moment,
With the trees as my witness,
I choose to give up my life to find yours.
And nothing is the same since you resided in my
heart. (4x)
And I am changed by being where the angels walked.
Singing holy is your name, holy is your name.
And I believe you are as real as the wind,
That brushes up against my heart,
And I know that your gaze is on me,
And you are smiling.
And right now in this moment,
I give up my life to find yours.
And I am changed by being where the angels walked.
Singing holy is your name, holy is your name.
And I believe you are as real as the wind,
That brushes up against my heart,
And I know that your gaze is on me,
And you are smiling.
And right now in this moment I choose
To give up my life to find yours. (2x)

Katie's First Journal Entry
(Written by Katie on March 28, 1995)

This was Katie's first journal entry when she was just 8 years old. She had a heart-shaped diary and on the inside cover she wrote a BIG warning to her older brother, Brian. "Don't even think about it, Brian!" was her message, just in case a curious older brother tried to read her entries to follow. Her first writing was dated March 28, 1995, which happens to be the same date 11 years later she would go to be with the Lord.

Katie wrote: "Dear God, I love you very much. You are very, nice, nice, nice, nice, good and all those things."

Her next entry later that year was: "Dear God, thank you for Jesus for dying on the cross for me. You are great. I enjoyed going to church today. Thank you for everything, for the gift of life. You are my favorite person in the world. I love you so, so, so, so much. You know all about my life. I hope I can live for you every day of my life. I like the world. But you know I can't wait to get to heaven. I hope I continue to live for you, Lord.

Please! Guide me through the troubles of the world. The only heart I want to have is a heart that helps others. I love chapel, and I think it brings me closer to you! I love singing praises. You are number one in my life. I can have joy, love Jesus-others-and you. Well, Katie signing off now. Bye."

Katie's Testimony
(Written by Katie at Rockford Master's Commission in the Fall of 2005)

I've always known that God had a special call on my life. When I was really young, a missions video was played at church, during which a heart kept beating as images flashed across the screen of starving children. The heart-beat stopped, and the missionary said that during the time of that video, people had died without ever hearing about Jesus. My mom saw tears in my eyes.

The closer I got to God, the more I felt disconnected with the "world," so I tried everything I could to be like everyone else. But it never seemed to be enough.

I was sinking fast. By my sophomore year, I didn't want to live anymore. I went to counseling and got on anti-depressants, but I felt dead inside. Nothing seemed to be able to fill the void inside of me.

But God didn't give up on me.

I learned about my youth group going on a missions trip to Portugal, and I knew that God wanted me to go. While there, I began to remember my first love. I was able to see firsthand that God is at work everywhere. And through everyone's prayers, God pulled me from the pit of depression.

After the trip, I went to a local college's open house, during which God showed me images of kids who wouldn't be helped if I went to that school as a writer. God brought to remembrance the Sunday school lesson about how Amy Carmichael rescued girls from India from prostitution.

I know that this is what God has called me to do.

"Heaven"
(Written by Katie in October 2005)

God, I want to follow in your footsteps. I see this image in my head of sand and a beach and me, just holding your hand, walking beside you, and you holding my face to your heart and saying, "It's gonna be okay," and wiping my tears, and picking me up and throwing me into the air and we could run through fields of daisies and you'd make one for me and I'd tickle you and fall into the grass laughing and I'd kiss you on the cheek and say, "I love you, Daddy." There are things about me that only you know. I don't have to bend my personality to fit other people's. I just need to know that I'm doing what you want. It doesn't matter what anybody thinks of me because I am unique to you. I'm lovely in your eyes. I'm your bride to be. You don't care if I wear make-up or straighten my hair. You are a toothpaste God, a getting ready in the morning

God, a sit by my bed and read me bedtime stories God, a Winnie-the-Pooh watching God, a caring God, a teddy bear God I can snuggle with at night, a sunshine God I think about first thing in the morning, a mosaic-tile God that I can think about when I step on the different colors, a sidewalk God who goes for walks with me, an endless God who always keeps giving, an eternal God.

I think heaven's gonna be <u>a lot</u> like childhood. There will be innocence. There will be kickball. There will be big slides that run down mansions. There will be neighborhood cook-outs and Jesus will be the fireworks. We will all turn our eyes to Him. It will be a little like the Fourth of July when me and Bethany would play for hours in the sun and go swimming and run around. You are the sparklers. God, you are sensational. It will be like the morning of Christmas when I would wake up the house because my stomach was gnawing itself and jumping because I was so excited. It will be like a wedding ceremony—the elation after the bride says I do and they kiss. It will be open and real. There will be hippie skirts and sunshine, and **I think the houses will be made of glass so we can all see each other because there will be nothing to hide—no barriers.** I think there will be different colors than here. God will be the main attraction, and perhaps we'll want to do nothing less than worship Him.

When I get to heaven, God, I want to lay at your feet and listen to your words and hear your breathing. I want to hold your warm, fleshy hand and kiss you a billion times for what you've done. I will hold you for a moment longer. It will be like the feeling Charlie gets when he found the golden ticket! Yet, nothing will compare to it—to seeing your face. I think it will be lovely. Your eyes will sparkle and your smile will have lines that raise to your eyes, and I'll just be able to feel your love for me by being near you, and I'll remember all the promises you had for me since I was a little girl, all the whispers you spoke in my softest dream, all the hope you instilled in me, the purpose, laying your hand on me when I went to sleep, letting me know in my deepest heart that you had a great purpose for my life. I want to follow that. I want to walk in that.

I remember when I lost it, and I turned to the world's purpose for me and how sad I felt, and I remember when I had to earn your love and how miserable I felt. But now I know that that sadness, that misery, that loneliness, that entrapment was me missing you. Our talks, our connection, our love.

You are a perfect sonnet, an impressed song that flows out of someone's life, the musical undertones. You are like a perfectly-sharpened pencil, a nightly walk between husband and wife, a shepherd's crook, all the deep things inside of me, someone's favorite sundae, a time apart from everyone else to listen to the crickets, you are the sunset. You are the freedom of letting go of the rope thread and falling into your arms jumping to you. Engagement rings and sunsets, princesses and fairy tales, marshmallows and spaghetti.

The cross, you are the suffering, too. You know the pain of separations, of loneliness, of not being understood, of not being approved by other people and, Jesus, you worked through that and so can I with your help. I am nothing on my own. But with you, all things are possible. I don't have to be like anyone else. Our relationship is unique and beautiful and you are my best friend and nothing could ever change that and somehow I can't comprehend how you are my Father and King yet friend and lover. You have seduced me. I admit it! Good job! You have won my love—but I want to give it all to you and not just some of it. I want it to be pure for you because you deserve my all. If a bride cares more about what family thinks, what friends think, than what husband thinks, then their relationship is already imbalanced. God, I want to be a good bride for you and this only through the grace of God—not my own works. And sometimes I think that I miss you more than words can say, which is weird cuz I've never seen you face to face, but I still miss you. I know I was meant to live with you forever. You are awesome, and your love is astounding. And I won't let anyone hold me back.

Everything I do today, I do it for you. And I <u>accept</u> your grace. When I fail, you don't condemn me. In fact, you expected it. You planned for it and that's why you sent your Son—not for perfect people but for imperfect people. By your grace, I am being perfected into more like you. You are refining me. You are taking all the excess weight off the ship at sea so I can really sail, throwing sandbags out of hot air balloons so I can soar with you. Your love is intimate and it changes me and I can't comprehend it. You're real. You made the heaven and earth and yet you love me. Wow, God, that's awesome. You're awesome and so cool and I love you and I'm yours. **Let's go for a picnic.**

Love, Your daughter,
Katie

"Gossip"
(Written by Katie in October 2005)

"The words of a gossip are like choice morsels; they go down to a man's inmost parts." (Proverbs 18:8)

"Without wood a fire goes out; without gossip a quarrel dies down." (Proverbs 26:20)

I, as a follower of Jesus, pledge that this year, I will not gossip about anyone here at Rockford Masters Commission or at home, nor listen to gossip. I will either change the subject or walk away. I realize that God wants our class to be united, so we cannot be "biting and devouring each other." Instead, I choose that in my conversations, I will lift my brothers and sisters in Christ up, not tear them down. I will abide by the Matthew 18 principle in which, if I have even the slightest problem with my brother or sister, I will go directly to them instead of asking other people if I should or getting their input on the situation. I will vent any issue I have with another person directly to God, realizing that if I have a problem with someone and share it with someone else (even if the motives are good), it then becomes the other person's problem and creates discord. **Gossip is a fire that fuels itself.** I realize that if there is a serious problem, I can talk directly to my discipleship director. I realize also that the "I could say this in front of the person, so it's okay" mentality is not gonna cut it because it justifies unproductive conversations.

"Before leaving for Master's"
(Written by Katie on September 21, 2005)

This is my hot pursuit for you, God. You pursued me for so long. Now it's my turn to pursue you in the hopes that I might find you, though you are not far from any one of us. Now my heart's desire be only for you, God. You are all that matters. Help me to put aside any distractions. Help me to seek you first, and everything else will be added, instead of doing it the other way around. Help me to have a heart more for other people than myself and to encourage others the way they have encouraged me. Help me to know how you always answer my prayers. Prepare my heart, God. Keep my attitudes in check. See if there is any offensive way in me, and lead me in the way everlasting. **I can't wait to spend eternity with you.** Please help me to put everything in perspective. You are all that matters. You are all I want. You love me so much and care about me and it is good. **I'm yours for the rest of my life, as long as you give me breath.** Give me the strength to take up my cross every day. Love, Your child, Katie

"What You Mean to Me"
(Written by Katie in the Summer of 2005)

I don't deserve this–any of this;
I don't deserve to wake up to a solitary beam
Of sunlight warming my soul.
To be able to feel a melodic heartbeat
Pulsing slowly, as water's waves
Speaking of your forgiveness forever.

To listen quietly the sweet foretelling of your soul
To feel my name spoken in every twilight
Every breath the dusk exhales after a forever-long day.

You are too good to me,
And I can't comprehend all the ways in which you
love me;
Your beauty is in every thought,
Every whisper,
In every silence that cannot be contained, even by the
water's depths.
You are there.
And though you have a million other children, I'm still
special to you.

Who...
Are you?
Is like you?
Can come to your throne room?

Surely not I, Lord. For you are too holy
And I am mere man. My life is but a breath.

When...
Will I trace your face for the first time?
Will your grace run dry?

You tell me never
And I don't know how this can be.

But I believe
That you are truer than the deepest hue of scarlet
That dances on the sunset.

Light reflected down to me, shining like prisms in precious gems
Upon those faces of those you love.

How do you love me, my God?
Where can I go that you are not?

I could never love you this way–
The way you love me, though I try,

I make excuses and I forget you
And I think too much–that I'm okay without you
sometimes
That I already know all there is to know about you.
I don't take you seriously.

And I forget you. I don't try to
It just happens, no matter how hard I will against it.
In this mortal body, my spirit cries for deliverance.

So today, maybe I'll wrap a flag around me,
Or pray for blurred faces of a magazine that need you.
Today, I'll try to love you,
To somehow express the ways in which I love you
Though these things you must already know.

Lord, sometimes I wonder what would happen
If everyone took you seriously.

"Dear God" Letter
(Written by Katie in her first week at RMC in September 2005 and opened and read by our family at her would-be graduation from RMC in June 2006)

Dear God, I love you so much. Thank you for taking me so far with you. I know that there is a long way to go, but we'll go there together, so everything will be okay. God, I'm very nervous about being here. It's hard leaving everything behind, but I know and am reminded that Christ did the same thing. Please help me this year to draw closer to you—so close that I can feel it. In this year, I don't want to do things halfheartedly or be casual about you. I want to give you my all this year and I know it's gonna take a fight. God, I want you to invade my life and my heart and take out all of the areas that are soiled, heal those that are broken. I pray this year that I will get rid of the fear of man and the constant aching for acceptance. Instead, I long to find my contentment and acceptance solely in you. Help me to be obedient to you and give you everything right away, instead of you having to take things away. Lord, I need you to be with me now. I pray that this year I would begin to accept your unfailing love for myself and others—that I would share the love you've shown my freely. Dear God, teach me things about you this year. Help me to get over any perfection-minded thinking and for your grace to simply be enough for me.

I pray that I would accept your grace. Also, God, please help me to be a giver, even if I don't get anything back. Lord, I want to be like Christ and I can't do this on my own. Teach me to be humble, I pray. May I always keep in mind that I am just a pen and you are the hand, and I can only be really used if you write with me. Otherwise, I am useless. Thank you for taking me here. I pray that you would help me to learn surrender, to learn your heart, to know you by heart. **Help me to follow your desires for my life, not mine, even if it means never getting married and dedicating my life and missionary work solely to you.** You desire obedience better than sacrifice. May my heart be obedient to your voice and not afraid of what others think this year. Help me to get over that. Help me to know how you really feel about me and not be lacking in self-worth because I think I don't measure up, because I know I always measure up to you, because you made me. Help me to think of the ministry you've called me to not as a burden or a sacrifice, but a joyous opportunity to give back what you've given me—to say thank you. Point your finger on my heart, I pray. Mold me, literally, into the woman of God that you want me to be. I feel as if we're on the verge of something and it's very exciting but it's also going to be challenging. My heart's desire is solely for you. May I put my whole heart into this program. Convict me. Test me. Mold me. Change me. Use me. Love me. Take me to where I never thought

I could go. Help me to be nicer to people, even if they seem annoying, because you love them. Help me to treat people the way you would were you in the situation. Even if kindness is "abused" by the world's standards, may I keep focused that I have a reward in heaven I'm working toward, not material wealth that quickly fades, and not to uphold a high opinion of myself so people think I am a good Christian. Help me to have more of a servant's heart and be less selfish—to give and give, and trust that you'll give back. Strengthen my faith, I pray. Help me to believe, to know you're real, and pray that way. May I see people as you see them. May I love you more. May I open up more and figure out that I can never quite figure out your love. **May my testimony bring me and others closer to you every time I say it.** Help me to find you here, to be more real. God, help me to live day by day instead of always worrying about what might happen, because all I have is now. Remind me of heaven and hell daily, I pray. Help me to be sensitive to your voice and not preoccupied with the logic, because how logical was it for Noah to build an ark? Make your word *rhema* to me, I pray. Make it apply, Lord, I pray. Help me to lay my life down, to be an unnamed hero, to not hog the spotlight but just be happy serving you. I need help with that. Help the people back home, I pray. Help the entire youth group to draw close to you. Help my parents and family. Help me, finally, to love the Lord my God with everything in me, and when

I get selfish, to love my neighbor <u>as myself</u>, and find out what this really means. I am yours for the next 9 months. Help me to hold nothing back. Take it all. Don't go easy on me. Don't let me quit. When I fall, I pray that you would pick me back up. Help me to think of the cross when I get weary. Help me to know that the sufferings of this present time are not worthy to be compared with the glory that will be revealed in us. Help me to find out new things about you every day. Help me to be able to resist the attacks of the enemy. Help me to love you more and to really fall in love with you this year. I give it all.

Love,

Katie

Graduation Letter
(Read at Katie and Wendi's Would-Be Graduation from RMC in June 2006; Written by Members of RMC Staff & Students)

We all remember the day in September when we stepped through the door to RMC, not knowing quite what to expect, but we knew there would be a change. So under God's direction, we proceeded to rearrange our lives, praying we'd never be the same. However we'd never expect all that would entail. They said we'd become a family, little did we know how true that was. Today we remember what we couldn't in September—all that God has done in the past nine months. But today we have to remember it without Katie and Wendi standing next to us.

These girls personified lives of change from the inside out, both overcomers, both conquerors, both victorious. We had watched them grow, without a doubt they were both different than they had been that very first day in September. Let's face it, they were both just different! Wendy's cups, tough questions, musicals, miss-matched shoes, laughing brown eyes, wild curly hair, basketball drills, and amped up ukuleles.

Both had smiles that gleamed, but with an underlying smirk that hinted at their constant mischief. Wendi's big brown eyes softened any trickery, and Katie's soft, sweet voice personified love, faith and devotion. The source of their joy can be traced to the secret places in which they found God. Under a pew, in the basement, in closets or corners, dancing and singing, and in every simple and beautiful thing, they met with God. Wendi and Katie both loved God with intensity; so deeply that they would keep much undiscovered by man; fully known by God alone.

Iron marks, shoes, laughter, adventure, silliness, yet all seriousness...they left us all so much. Today we celebrate our friends. Katie embodied the abundant life God promised to all of us. To her we say—you are a shooting star of inspiration that we treasure. Wendi embodied a beautiful mix of determination and exuberance. To her we say—you inspire us to move with the dance God has given us.

We recall that day in March when things just seemed to stop…but the reality is that we aren't finishing without them, they are simply starting the final phase of life before us. And as much as we miss them, that fits who they are. It has been said that to love is to receive a glimpse of Heaven. Wendi, Katie, because of your love for God, for others, and for life, we trust that when you entered Heaven and approached the Throne, you found it a familiar place. We will meet you there. Thanks for giving us a glimpse of Heaven in the love you lived. Let's walk on together. Hallelujah!

CPSIA information can be obtained
at www.ICGtesting.com
Printed in the USA
BVHW011555190622
639756BV00001B/3